# Plant Based Diet:

The Perfect Plan To Reset Your Body And Boost Your Energy. A Kick-Start Guide To Cook And Live Your Best. Easy Meatless Recipes For Sane Nutrition Also Good For The Environment.

Table of Contents

**Chapter 3.        Soup Recipes**

*Hibiscus Latte*

*Turmeric Eggnog*

**Conclusion**

# Introduction

Plant-based diet can vary from one person to another. However, the foundational idea is that we try to avoid processed food as much as possible and choose to use what we receive from the beautiful planet that we live in. By that, I mean the incredible ingredients derived from the earth. In essence, plant-based diet comes with a few benefits.

Plant-based diet avoids using processed foods as much as possible.

There are no animal products in the diet.

The categories that are majorly included are vegetables, fruits, seeds and nuts, legumes, whole grains, and herbs and spices.

The diet tries to limit the use of sugar, wheat-flour, and oil as much as possible.

It focuses on the quality of food, mostly utilizing locally or farm-produced organic foods

An important thing to remember here is that there are minimally processed foods included in the plant-based diet, such as non-dairy milk, tofu, and whole-wheat paste, to name a few. Overall, we aim to keep processed foods where they belong: on supermarket shelves, not in our refrigerators.

When people look at the list of foods that come in a plant-based diet, they are often focused on how little we have to work on. However, that is probably due to the fact that many of the meat options have suddenly been removed. It feels as though a major part of the diet has been excluded due to it. How can life be fun without a nice steak? What can we do without chicken wings? Is there anything that can be done without a delicious fish?

In reality, there are numerous ingredients that you can work with. Additionally, the fun is not just in the ingredients but how we prepare them. The growing demand has seen a rise in people trying out new recipes and mashing up ingredients in interesting ways. Have you heard of smoothies that contain cayenne pepper? Sounds pretty exciting, doesn't it? We are going to look at such wonderful and delicious recipes along with so many more dishes that use wholesome and natural ingredients.

People who follow plant-based diets and consume a wide variety of fruits, vegetables and pulses are likely to find it easier to achieve their target of five days.

Some people are doing it; some people are talking about it, but there is still a lot of confusion about what a whole plant-based diet actually entails. Since we split food into their macronutrients: sugars, proteins, and fats, most of us are uncertain about nutrition. What if we were able to put these macronutrients back together again in order to free your mind from confusion and stress? The secret here is simplicity.

# Chapter 1.      The Basics Of A Plant-Based Diet

What Is A Plant-Based Diet?

Whole foods are foods that come from the earth unprocessed. Now, on a whole food plant-based diet, we eat some minimally processed foods like whole bread, whole wheat pasta, tofu, nondairy milk, and some nuts and seed butter. All of these are fine as long as they are handled to a minimum. So here are the different categories:

Legumes (basically lentils and beans) of whole grains.

Fruits and vegetables

Nuts and seeds (including nut butter)

Herbs and spices

All categories mentioned above constitute an entire diet based on plants. Directions them is where the fun comes in; how to season and cook them; and how to mix and match to give them great flavor and variety in your meals. In this book, there are chapters devoted to plant-based recipes that can give you an idea of what you can easily whip up in your kitchen or the special meals that you can make for your friends. So long, so you regularly eat these foods, you will forever forget about sugars, protein, and fat.

Now, some may say, "Well, I can't eat soy," "I don't like tofu," and so on. Well, the beauty of an entire diet based on food plants is that if you don't like some food, like soy, in this case, you don't have to eat it. In a whole plant-based diet, it is not a necessary component. Instead of barley, you can get brown rice, quinoa instead of wheat; I'm sure you catch the drift right now. It really does not matter. Only find the right thing for you.

Just because you decided to adopt a plant-based diet lifestyle, that doesn't mean it's a healthy diet. Plant-based diets have a fair share of junk and other unhealthy foods, case and point, regular veggie pizza, and non-dairy ice cream consumption. Staying healthy requires you to eat healthy foods—even in a dietary setting, based on plants.

A few words that fly around are a similar eating style, but they're both distinct. That doesn't mean you're going to have to tag yourself to adhere to that way of eating; these words define various ways of eating to help you understand what types of food choices are in a particular class. This analysis can also help you understand how a diet based on a crop blends into the larger picture.

Plant-based: This way of eating is based on berries, vegetables, rice, legumes, nuts, and seeds with few or no foods of animal origin. The plant-based diet is preferably a vegan diet with some versatility in the intermediate stages, with the intention of becoming 100% plant-based over time.

Vegan: It describes someone who eats nothing from an animal, be it fish, fowl, rodents, or insects. Vegans refrain from animal meats as well as from other animal-made foods (such as milk and honey). They also often abstain from buying, wearing or using any kind of animal products (e.g., leather).

Fruit: it represents a vegan diet consisting primarily of fruit.

Raw vegan: This is an uncooked vegan diet that often includes dehydrated foods. Vegetarian: Sometimes, this plant-based diet includes milk and eggs.

Flexitarian: This plant-based diet includes the occasional meat or fish consumption. I like to call it "a little bit of this and a little bit of it" — said, of course, without judgment!

Why You Need To Cut Back On Processed And Animal-Based Products

You've probably heard that fast food is bad for you over and over again. "Avoid preservatives; avoid processed foods;" but no one really gives you any real or solid information about why they should be avoided and why they are dangerous. So let's break it down so you can fully understand why these guilty culprits should be stopped.

They have huge addictive properties

We have a strong tendency as humans to be addicted to certain foods, but the fact is that it is not our fault entirely. Practically all of the unhealthy foods we indulge in activate our dopamine neurotransmitter brains from time to time. It makes the brain feel "healthy," but this is for only a short time. This also creates a tendency toward addiction; that's why somebody will always find themselves going back to another candy bar—even if they don't really need it. Through cutting the stimulus entirely, you will stop all this.

They are loaded sugar and high fructose corn syrup

Processed and animals based products are loaded with sugars and high fructose corn syrup with a nutritional value that is close to zero. More and more studies are now showing what many people have always suspected; that genetically modified foods cause inflammation of the gut, which in turn makes it more difficult for the body to absorb essential nutrients. The downside of your body, from muscle loss and brain fog to fat gain, cannot be stressed enough if you fail to properly absorb essential nutrients.

They are loaded with refined carbohydrates

Processed foods are loaded with refined carbs and products based on animals. Yes, it is a fact that carbs are needed in your body to provide energy to perform body functions. However, the refining of carbs eliminates the essential nutrients; it eliminates the whole grain component by refining whole grains. After refining, what you're left with is what's called "empty" carbs. By spiking blood sugar and insulin levels, these can have a negative impact on your metabolism.

They are loaded with artificial ingredients

Your body treats them as a foreign object when you consume artificial ingredients. They become an invader in essence. The body is not used to accept things like sucralose or artificial sweeteners. So, your body is doing the best it can. It triggers an immune response that reduces your resistance to disease, making you vulnerable. Otherwise, your body's focus and energy on protecting your immune system could be diverted elsewhere.

They contain components that cause a hyper reward sense in your body

What this means is that they contain components such as monosodium glutamate (MSG), highfructose corn syrup components, and certain colors that can carve addictive properties. They are encouraging your body to receive a reward from it. For example, MSG is present in many prepackaged pastries. What this does is that to enjoy the taste, it stimulates your taste buds. Just by the way your brain communicates with your taste buds, it becomes psychological.

This reward-based system makes your body want more and more, putting you at a severe risk of over-consumption of calories. What about food from animals? The term "low quality" is often used to refer to plant proteins as they tend to have lower amounts of essential amino acids than animal proteins. What most people don't realize is that more essential amino acids can be harmful to their health. Now, let's discuss more on that.

Animal Protein Lacks Fiber

Most people end up displacing the plant protein they already had in their quest to load more animal protein. This is poor because, unlike plant protein, animal protein lacks fiber, antioxidants, and phytonutrients. Fiber deficiency in various communities and societies around the world is quite common. According to the Institute of Medicine, for instance, in the USA, the average adult absorbs only about 15 grams of fiber per day relative to the 38 grams required. Lack of adequate intake of dietary fiber is associated with increased risk of colon and breast cancer, as well as disease of Crohn, heart disease, and constipation.

Animal protein causes a spike in IGF-1

IGF-1 is the growth factor-1-like hormone insulin. It stimulates cell division and growth, which may sound good but also stimulates cancer cell growth. Therefore, higher blood levels of IGF-1 are associated with increased risk of cancer, malignancy, and proliferation. Animal protein causes phosphorus to increase

Animal protein contains high levels of phosphorus

By secreting a hormone called fibroblast growth factor 23 (FGF23), our bodies normalize the high levels of phosphorus. FGF23 was also found to cause irregular heart muscle enlargement—a risk factor in extreme cases of heart failure and even death.

Instead, given all the issues, the "high quality" of animal protein's aspect might be more appropriately described as "high risk." Like caffeine, which you will feel withdrawal symptoms after you completely cut it off, processed foods can be cut off immediately. Maybe the one thing you're going to lose is the comfort of not having to prepare every meal from scratch.

Plant-Based Diet Vs. Vegan

Mistaking a vegan diet for a plant-based diet is quite common for people or vice versa. Okay, although there are parallels between both diets, they are not quite the same. So let's really break it down quickly.

Vegan

A vegan diet is one that does not include products based on animals. This includes meat, dairy, eggs, and products or ingredients such as honey derived from animals. Someone who describes himself as a vegan carries this perspective into their daily lives. What this means is that they are not using or encouraging the use of clothing, boots, accessories, shampoos, and make-ups made from animal products. For example, wool, beeswax, leather, gelatin, silk, and lanolin are included. People's inspiration to live a vegan lifestyle also comes from an urge to stand up and fight animal mistreatment and bad animal ethical treatment, as well as to support animal rights.

Plant-Based Diet

On the other hand, an entire diet based on food plants shares a similarity with veganism in the sense that it does not also promote the dietary consumption of products based on animals. It covers eggs, meat, and dairy. What's more, unlike the vegan diet, the diet does not include processed foods, white flour, oils, and refined sugars. The aim here is to create a diet of unprocessed vegetables, herbs, whole grains, nuts, seeds and legumes that are minimally processed.

The health benefits it offers are often guided by full-food plant-based diet followers. It is a diet that has very little to do with calorie restriction or macro counting, but mostly with disease prevention and reversal.

Getting Started On A Whole Food Plant-Based Diet

Common misconceptions among many people—even some in the health and fitness industry is that anyone who switches to a plant-based diet becomes super healthy automatically. There are plenty of plant-based junk foods out there, such as non-dairy ice cream and frozen veggie pizza, which can really destroy your health goals if you consume them all the time. The only way you can achieve health benefits is to commit to healthy foods. On the other hand, in keeping you inspired, these plant-based snacks play a role. In moderation, sparingly and in small bits, they should be consumed. There's a section dedicated to giving suggestions on plant-based snacks that you can cook up at home, as you'll see later in this book. So, this is how you get started on a whole plant-based recipe without further ado.

Decide What a Plant-Based Diet Means for You

The first step is to make a decision to structure how your plant-based diet will look, and it will help you transition from your current dietary outlook. This is really personal, something that varies from person to person. While some people choose not to tolerate any animal products at all, some occasionally make do with tiny bits of milk or meat. Deciding what and how you want your plant-based diet to look like is really up to you. The most important thing is that you must make a large majority of your diet from whole plant-based foods.

Understand What You Are Eating

Okay, now that you have taken the decision, your next step will require a great deal of analysis on your side. What do we meaning by this? Well, if this is your first time trying out the plantbased diet, you may be surprised by the number of foods that contain animal products, especially packaged foods. When shopping, you'll find yourself cultivating the habit of reading tags. This points out that many pre-packaged foods contain animal products, and if you only want to stick to plant products for your new diet, you need to keep a close eye on the labeling of the ingredients. Maybe you've decided to allow a certain amount of animal products in your diet; well, you're just going to have to watch out for foods filled with oils, sugars, salt, preservatives, and other items that might have an effect on your healthy diet.

Find Revamped Versions of Your Favorite Recipes

I'm sure you've got a number of favorite, not necessarily plant-based dishes. Leaving everything behind is typically the hardest part for most people. There's still a way to meet you halfway, though. Take some time to talk about those non-plant-based foods that you like. Think along the lines of flavor, texture, versatility, and so on; and look for swaps in the entire diet based on food plants that can fulfill what you're missing.

Build a Support Network

It's hard to build a new habit, but it doesn't have to be. Find some friends, or even family members, who are happy to be with you in this lifestyle. This will help you stay focused and inspired while also having a form of transparency and emotional support. You can do fun things like trying out and sharing with these friends new recipes or even hitting up restaurants that offer a variety of plant-based choices. You can even go a step further and look up local social media plant-based groups to help you expand your network of knowledge and support.

Valuable vegetables

You'll find a whole variety of vegetables that you'll really get to know quite well when eating plant-based veggies. If you're new to this, at the beginning, you're likely to stick to tried-andtrue, popular veggies because they're going to feel healthy. These vegetables are a good start:

Beets

Carrots

Kale

Parsley, basil, and other herbs

Spinach

Squash

Sweet potatoes

Fantastic fruits

We all love it! You need to get on this train if you haven't because the fruits are delicious; sweet; full of sugar, color, and beautiful vitamins; and so, so good for you.

Apples

Avocado

Bananas

Blueberries

Coconut

Mango

Pears

Pineapple

Raspberries

Strawberries

Wonderful whole grains

Consuming whole grains of good quality is a healthy part of a diet based on vegetables. Don't worry; you can still have your pastas and breads, but the key word here is "whole." You don't want the real thing to be polished or stored. When purchasing these items, make sure that the only ingredient is the grain itself. While it is possible to purchase proper whole grains in packaging from the shelf, make sure that you double-check the label to confirm that it is indeed a whole grain (and just a whole grain).

Brown rice

Brown-rice pasta

Quinoa Rolled oats

Sprouted-grain spelt bread

Lovable legumes

Learning to love beans on a plant-based diet is important because they are a great source of food, protein, and fuel. It may take you and your body a while to get used to them, but they will soon be your friends—especially when you find out how great it is to eat them in soups, salads, burgers, and other creative media. Here are some of the best things to begin with:

Black beans

Chickpeas

Kidney beans

Lentils

Split peas

Notable nuts and seeds

A decent handful of nuts is good. But the thing about eating them on a plant-based diet is to make sure they're unsalted, unoiled, and raw. You can feel free to eat them in moderation alongside your other wonderful plant-based foods as long as you enjoy them in their natural state. Here are the best to begin with:

Almonds

Cashews

Chia seeds

Flaxseeds

Hempseeds

Pumpkin seeds

Sunflower seeds

Walnuts

Mental resistance is one of the biggest challenges people face when they decide to take up a plant-based diet. In reality, maybe you think it's too hard, or it's just another diet that won't last or produce the results you're hoping for. Eating a plant-based diet isn't just a fad or something you're doing for weight loss or short-term outcomes. This book is about using plants as your fuel to lead a healthier lifestyle. You need to eat at the end of the day, so why not make your meals and snacks fibrous, delicious, and plant-loaded? I truly believe that with the information contained in this book, together with a keen interest in healthy living, you will discover that consuming a plant-based diet is not difficult and that anybody can

Mental resistance is one of the biggest challenges people face when they decide to take up a plant-based diet. In reality, maybe you think it's too hard, or it's just another diet that won't last or produce the results you're hoping for. Eating a plant-based diet isn't just a fad or something you're doing for weight loss or short-term outcomes. This book is about using plants as your fuel to lead a healthier lifestyle.

# Chapter 2.     Breakfast Recipes

## Chia Seed Smoothie

Servings: 3

Preparation Time: 5 Minutes

Calories: 477

Protein: 8 Grams

Fat: 29 Grams

Carbs: 57 Grams

Ingredients:

¼ Teaspoon Cinnamon

1 Tablespoon Ginger, Fresh & Grated

Pinch Cardamom

1 Tablespoon Chia Seeds

2 Medjool Dates, Pitted

1 Cup Alfalfa Sprouts

1 Cup Water

1 Banana

½ Cup Coconut Milk, Unsweetened

Directions:

Blend everything together until smooth.

## Mango Smoothie

Servings: 3

Preparation Time: 5 Minutes

Calories: 376

Protein: 5 Grams

Fat: 2 Grams

Carbs: 95 Grams

Ingredients:

1 Carrot, Peeled & Chopped

1 Cup Strawberries

1 Cup Water

1 Cup Peaches, Chopped

1 Banana, Frozen & sliced

1 Cup Mango, Chopped

Directions:

Blend everything together until smooth.

## Quinoa & Chocolate Bowl

Servings: 2

Preparation Time: 35 Minutes

Calories: 392

Protein: 12 Grams

Fat: 19 Grams

Carbs: 49 Grams

Ingredients:

1 Cup Quinoa

1 Cup Almond Milk, Unsweetened

1 Teaspoon Cinnamon

1 Banana

1 Cup Water

2-3 Tablespoons Cocoa Powder, Unsweetened

2 Tablespoons Almond Butter

1 Tablespoon Chia Seeds, Ground

2 Tablespoons Walnuts, Optional

¼ Cup Raspberries, Fresh

Directions:

Place your cinnamon, milk, water and quinoa in a pot, bringing it to a boil before turning it down to low heat to simmer. Cover, simmering for twenty-five to thirty minutes.

Puree your banana, mixing in your almond butter, flaxseed and cocoa powder.

Scoop a cup of quinoa into a bowl, and then top with pudding, raspberries and walnuts if you're using them before serving.

## Vegetable Hash

Servings: 4

Preparation Time: 35 Minutes

Calories: 273

Protein: 9 Grams

Fat: 11 Grams

Carbs: 39 Grams

Ingredients:

1 Tablespoon Sage Leaves, Chopped

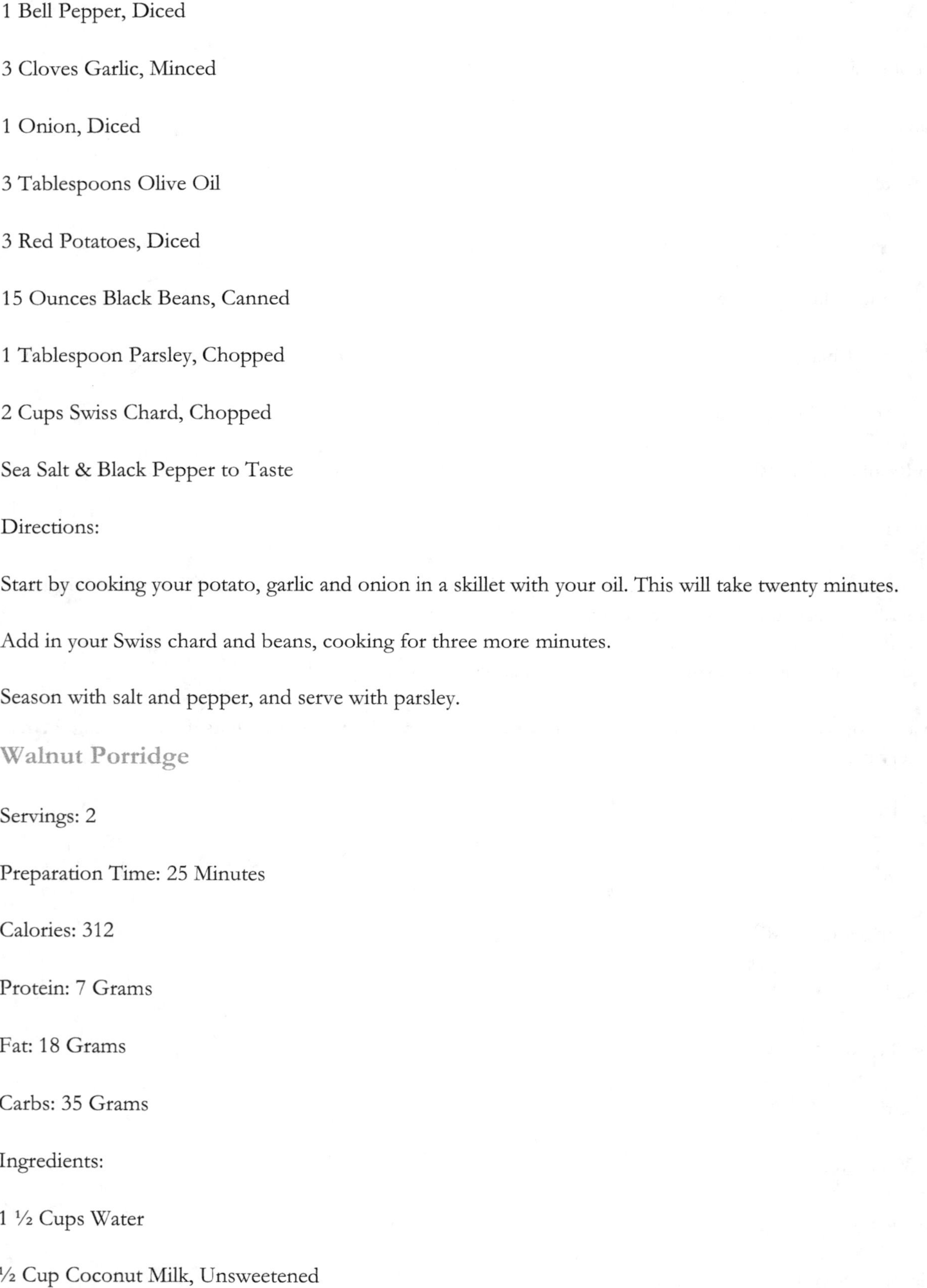

1 Bell Pepper, Diced

3 Cloves Garlic, Minced

1 Onion, Diced

3 Tablespoons Olive Oil

3 Red Potatoes, Diced

15 Ounces Black Beans, Canned

1 Tablespoon Parsley, Chopped

2 Cups Swiss Chard, Chopped

Sea Salt & Black Pepper to Taste

Directions:

Start by cooking your potato, garlic and onion in a skillet with your oil. This will take twenty minutes.

Add in your Swiss chard and beans, cooking for three more minutes.

Season with salt and pepper, and serve with parsley.

## Walnut Porridge

Servings: 2

Preparation Time: 25 Minutes

Calories: 312

Protein: 7 Grams

Fat: 18 Grams

Carbs: 35 Grams

Ingredients:

1 ½ Cups Water

½ Cup Coconut Milk, Unsweetened

1 Cup Teff, Whole Grain

½ Teaspoon Cardamom, Ground

1 Teaspoon Sea Salt, Fine

¼ Cup Walnuts, Chopped

1 Tablespoon Maple Syrup, Pure

Directions:

Start by combining your coconut oil and water, bringing it to a boil before stirring in your teff.

Add the cardamom, and then allow it to simmer for twenty minutes.

Mix in your walnuts and maple syrup before serving.

## Granola

Servings: 7

Preparation Time: 1 Hour 30 Minutes

Calories: 239

Protein: 6 Grams

Fat: 11 Grams

Carbs: 32 Grams

Ingredients:

½ Cup Maple Syrup, Pure

¼ Cup Coconut Oil

¾ Cup Coconut, Unsweetened & Shredded

1 Cup Almonds, Slivered

¾ Teaspoon Sea Salt, Fine

5 Cups Rolled Oats

Directions:

Start by heating your oven to 250, and then mix all of your ingredients together in a bowl.

Spread your granola out over two baking sheets, making sure it's spread out evenly.

Bake for an hour and fifteen minutes, but you'll need to stir every twenty minutes.

Allow it to cool before serving.

## Breakfast Cereal

Servings: 6

Preparation Time: 45 Minutes

Calories: 160

Protein: 3 Grams

Fat: 1.5 Grams

Carbs: 34 Grams

Ingredients:

¼ Tablespoon Butter

2 ¼ Cups Water

Honey to Taste

1 Teaspoon Cinnamon

1 Cup Brown Rice, Uncooked

½ Cup Raisins, Seedless

Directions:

Start by combining your cinnamon, raisins, rice, and butter in a saucepan before adding in your water. Bring it to a boil, and allow it to simmer while covered for forty minutes. Fluff with a fork.

Serve with honey.

# Fruity Oatmeal

Servings: 2

Preparation Time: 25 Minutes

Calories: 230

Protein: 4.6 Grams

Fat: 5.6 Grams

Carbs: 43.8 Grams

Ingredients:

½ Cup Apple Juice, Fresh & Frozen

½ Cup Oatmeal

½ Cup Water

3 Prunes, Diced

1 Apple, Small & Diced

4 Pecans, Diced

3 Apricots, Dehydrated, Dried & Diced

¼ Teaspoon Cinnamon

Directions:

Start by getting out a small saucepan and mix together your apple juice and water, bringing the mixture to a boil.

Add a half a cup of oatmeal, cooking for a minute. Add in your pecans, cinnamon and fruit pieces. Make sure to stir. If you want to make sure you have more vitamins, add in your fruit when your oatmeal is nearly cool.

# Pecan Pumpkin Spice Oatmeal

Preparation Time: 15 Minutes
Servings: 2

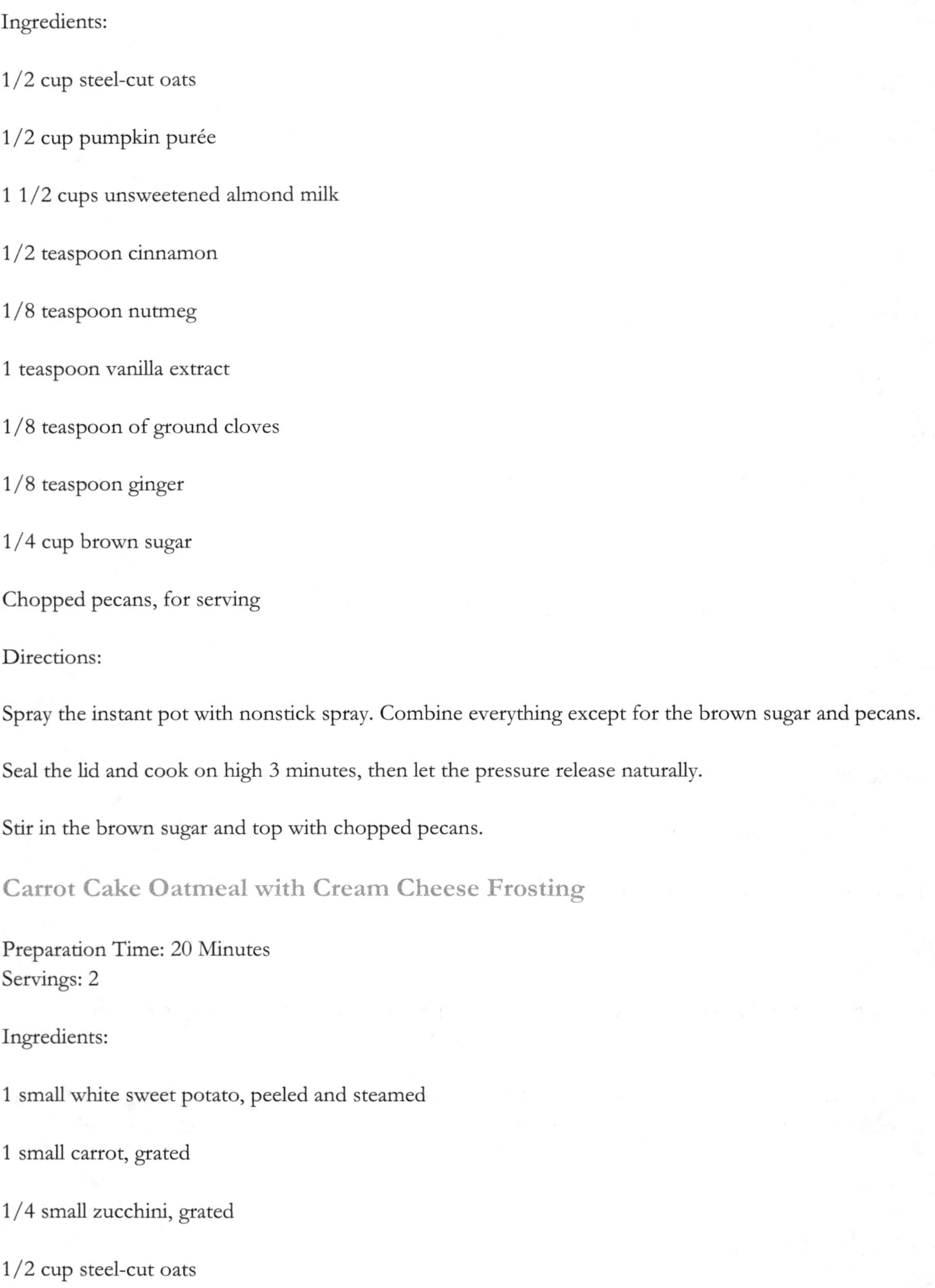

Ingredients:

1/2 cup steel-cut oats

1/2 cup pumpkin purée

1 1/2 cups unsweetened almond milk

1/2 teaspoon cinnamon

1/8 teaspoon nutmeg

1 teaspoon vanilla extract

1/8 teaspoon of ground cloves

1/8 teaspoon ginger

1/4 cup brown sugar

Chopped pecans, for serving

Directions:

Spray the instant pot with nonstick spray. Combine everything except for the brown sugar and pecans.

Seal the lid and cook on high 3 minutes, then let the pressure release naturally.

Stir in the brown sugar and top with chopped pecans.

## Carrot Cake Oatmeal with Cream Cheese Frosting

Preparation Time: 20 Minutes
Servings: 2

Ingredients:

1 small white sweet potato, peeled and steamed

1 small carrot, grated

1/4 small zucchini, grated

1/2 cup steel-cut oats

1 1/2 cups nondairy milk

1/2 teaspoon lemon juice

1/2 teaspoon apple cider vinegar

1/8 teaspoon of salt

1/8 teaspoon ground cloves

1/8 teaspoon nutmeg

1/2 teaspoon cinnamon

2 tablespoons brown sugar

2 tablespoons maple syrup

1 1/2 tablespoons coconut oil

1 tablespoon water

Directions:

To make the cream cheese frosting, puree half of the steamed sweet potato in a food processor. Add the maple syrup, water, coconut oil, lemon juice, and apple cider vinegar and puree until smooth. Add more sweet potato if the mixture is not thick enough.

Spray the instant pot with nonstick spray. Combine the rest of the ingredients, then seal the lid and cook on high 3 minutes.

Let the pressure release naturally. Add additional milk to the oatmeal if needed, and top each serving with a dollop of the cream cheese frosting.

## Chocolate Walnut Oatmeal

Preparation Time: 15 Minutes
Servings: 2

Ingredients:

1/2 cup steel-cut oats

2 tablespoons cocoa powder

1 teaspoon brown sugar

1 tablespoon agave nectar

1 teaspoon vanilla extract

1/2 cup unsweetened almond milk

1 1/2 cups water

Semi-sweet chocolate chips, for topping

Walnuts for topping

Directions:

Spray the instant pot with nonstick spray. Combine the oats, cocoa powder, water, vanilla, brown sugar, and agave nectar.

Cook on high 3 minutes, then let the pressure release naturally. Stir in the almond milk.

Top with chocolate chips and walnuts.

## Breakfast Burrito Filling

Preparation Time: 15 Minutes
Servings: 4

Ingredients:

15 ounces tofu, drained and crumbled

1/2 cup water

1 clove garlic, minced

1/2 bell pepper, chopped

1/2 teaspoon chili powder

1/4 teaspoon chipotle chili powder

1/4 teaspoon sriracha sauce

1 teaspoon lime juice

Salt and pepper, to taste

1/4 cup shredded vegan cheddar cheese, for serving

Warm tortillas, for serving

Salsa, for serving

Directions:

Combine all the ingredients in the instant pot. Seal the lid and cook on high 4 minutes, then let the pressure release naturally.

If the mixture is too wet, drain off some of the water. Stir in the cheese to melt it. Serve wrapped warm tortillas with salsa.

## Tofu Breakfast Custard and Potatoes

Preparation Time: 25 Minutes
Servings: 4

Ingredients:

12 ounces frozen hash browns

1 shallot, chopped

2 tablespoons vegan chicken-flavored bouillon

10 ounces silken tofu

1/2 cup shredded vegan cheddar cheese

1/2 cup nondairy milk

1/4 teaspoon onion powder

1/8 teaspoon garlic powder

1/2 teaspoon seasoned salt

1/4 teaspoon freshly ground pepper

1 tablespoon olive oil

Hot sauce, for serving

Directions:

Puree the tofu, milk, bouillon, garlic powder, onion powder and seasoned salt in a food processor.

Heat the oil in the instant pot on the sauté setting and cook the shallot for 3 minutes.

Spread the hash browns on top of the cooked shallots, and top with the cheese. Pour the tofu puree over the top, then sprinkle with fresh ground pepper.

Cook on high 5 minutes, then quick release the pressure.

The tofu mixture should be a jiggly custard texture. If it is too moist, return the instant pot to the sauté setting and cook longer with the lid on but vented.

Serve with hot sauce!

## Apple and Sausage French Toast Casserole

Preparation Time: 25 Minutes
Servings: 4

Ingredients:

4 links vegan breakfast sausages, chopped into coins

2 apples, peeled and chopped

Juice of 1/2 lemon

Zest of 1/2 lemon

1/2 loaf whole wheat bread, chopped into cubes

1 1/2 cups water

1 teaspoon vanilla extract

3 tablespoons unsweetened applesauce

1/2 teaspoon cinnamon

1 tablespoon olive oil

Maple syrup, for serving

Directions:

Heat olive oil in the instant pot using the sauté setting. Add the sausage and cook for 10 minutes.

Add the water, applesauce, vanilla extract, lemon juice, and cinnamon to the instant pot. Add the apples, then the bread cubes. Push the bread down to make sure it is all coated with the mixture.

Seal the lid and cook on high 4 minutes, then let the pressure release naturally. Dust with powdered sugar and lemon zest and serve.

## Granola.

Preparation Time: 25 Minutes
Servings: 8 cups

Ingredients:

5 cups old-fashioned rolled oats

1 cup slivered blanched almonds

⅔ cup pure maple syrup

½ cup wheat germ

½ cup unsweetened shredded coconut

½ cup sunflower seeds

½ cup golden raisins or sweetened dried cranberries

½ cup chopped dates or dried apricots

¼ cup vegetable oil

¼ cup packed light brown sugar

3 tablespoons water

1 teaspoon pure vanilla extract

Directions:

Spray the Instant Pot insert with cooking spray and set to high.

Add the maple syrup, oil, water, sugar, and vanilla.

In a bowl combine the oats, wheat germ, almonds, sunflower seeds, coconut, and dates.

Mix the oats into the syrup mix in the Instant Pot.

Seal and cook on Meat for 12 minutes.

Release the pressure and cook with the lid open until your granola is crisp.

## Granola Oats.

Preparation Time: 50 Minutes
Servings: 4

Ingredients:

4½ cups water

1¼ cups old-fashioned rolled oats or steel-cut oats

1 cup granola

1½ teaspoons ground cinnamon

½ teaspoon salt

Directions:

Lightly oil your Instant Pot insert with cooking spray.

Combine the oats, water, cinnamon, and salt.

Seal and cook on Stew for 40 minutes.

Release the pressure naturally and stir in the granola.

36. Spiced Apple Oats.

Preparation Time: 50 Minutes
Servings: 4

Ingredients:

3 cups water

2 cups apple juice

2 apples, peeled, cored, and chopped

1¼ cups steel-cut oats

½ cup golden raisins or dried cranberries

¼ cup packed light brown sugar or granulated natural sugar, or more to taste

1 tablespoon ground flaxseed

1 teaspoon ground cinnamon

½ teaspoon salt

Directions:

Lightly oil your Instant Pot insert with cooking spray.

Combine the ingredients.

Seal and cook on Stew for 40 minutes.

## PB&J Oats.

Preparation Time: 50 Minutes
Servings: 6

Ingredients:

5½ cups water

1½ cups steel-cut oats

½ cup strawberry jam

½ cup creamy peanut butter, at room temperature

1 teaspoon ground cinnamon

¾ teaspoon salt

Directions:

Lightly oil your Instant Pot insert with cooking spray.

Combine the oats, water, cinnamon, and salt.

Seal and cook on Stew for 40 minutes.

Release the pressure naturally and stir in the peanut butter and jam.

## Choco-Coco Milk Shake

Preparation Time: 25 MIN

Servings:  1

Ingredients:

½ cup whole milk

1 tbsp cocoa powder

1 packet Stevia, or more to taste

1 tbsp coconut flakes, unsweetened

1 cup water

1 tbsp coconut oil

Directions:

Add all ingredients in blender.

Blend until smooth and creamy.

Serve and enjoy.

Nutrition:

Calories per serving: 263; Carbohydrates: 22.7g; Protein: 4.8g; Fat: 20.65g; Sugar: 14.7g; Sodium: 75mg; Fiber: 2.1g

## Nutty Choco Milk Shake

Preparation Time: 25 MIN

Servings:  1

Ingredients:

¼ cup whole milk

1 tbsp cocoa powder

1 packet Stevia, or more to taste

¼ cup pecans

1 ½ cups water

1 tbsp macadamia oil

Directions:

Add all ingredients in blender.

Blend until smooth and creamy.

Serve and enjoy.

Nutrition:

Calories per serving: 358; Carbohydrates: 15.5g; Protein: 5.1g; Fat: 34.0g; Sugar: 8.9g; Sodium: 33mg; Fiber: 4g

## Gritty Choco Milk Shake

Preparation Time: 25 MIN

Servings:  1

Ingredients:

¼ cup whole milk

1 tbsp cocoa powder

1 packet Stevia, or more to taste

1 tbsp chia seeds

1 tbsp hemp seeds

1 tbsp flaxseed

1 ½ cups water

1 tbsp Flaxseed oil

Directions:

Add all ingredients in blender.

Blend until creamy yet still gritty. If preferred, blend until smooth.

Serve and enjoy.

Nutrition:

Calories per serving: 363; Carbohydrates: 22.8g; Protein: 8.9g; Fat: 29.4g; Sugar: 8.3g; Sodium: 42mg; Fiber: 10.1g

## Creamy Choco Shake

Preparation Time: 25 MIN

Servings:  1

Ingredients:

½ cup heavy cream

2 tbsps cocoa powder

1 packet Stevia, or more to taste

1 cup water

Directions:

Add all ingredients in blender.

Blend until smooth and creamy.

Serve and enjoy.

Nutrition:

Calories per serving: 435; Carbohydrates: 10.6g; Protein: 4.6g; Fat: 45.5g; Sugar: 3.5g; Sodium: 52mg; Fiber: 4g

## Raspberry-Choco Shake

Preparation Time: 25 MINUTES

Servings:  1

Ingredients:

½ cup heavy cream, liquid

1 tbsp cocoa powder

1 packet Stevia, or more to taste

¼ cup raspberries

1 ½ cups water

Directions:

Add all ingredients in blender.

Blend until smooth and creamy.

Serve and enjoy.

Nutrition:

Calories per serving: 438; Carbohydrates: 11.1g; Protein: 3.8g; Fat: 45.0g; Sugar: 4.8g; Sodium: 54mg; Fiber: 3.6g

## Strawberry-Choco Shake

Preparation Time: 25 MINUTES

Servings:  1

Ingredients:

½ cup heavy cream, liquid

1 tbsp cocoa powder

1 packet Stevia, or more to taste

½ cup strawberry, sliced

1 tbsp coconut flakes, unsweetened

1 ½ cups water

Directions:

Add all ingredients in blender.

Blend until smooth and creamy.

Serve and enjoy.

Nutrition:

Calories per serving: 470; Carbohydrates: 15.7g; Protein: 4.1g; Fat: 46.4g; Sugar: 8.9g; Sodium: 69mg; Fiber: 3.6g

## Almond Choco Shake

Preparation Time: 25 MINUTES

Servings:  1

Ingredients:

½ cup heavy cream, liquid

1 tbsp cocoa powder

1 packet Stevia, or more to taste

½ cup almonds, chopped

1 ½ cups water

Directions:

Soak almonds in water for at least 30 minutes.

Then, add all ingredients in blender.

Blend until smooth and creamy.

Serve and enjoy.

Nutrition:

Calories per serving: 485; Carbohydrates: 15.7g; Protein: 11.9g; Fat: 45.9g; Sugar: 3.8g; Sodium: 31mg; Fiber: 7.4g

## Gritty and Nutty Shake

Preparation Time: 25 MINUTES

Servings: 1

Ingredients:

¼ cup heavy cream, liquid

½ tbsp cocoa powder

1 packet Stevia, or more to taste

¼ cup almonds, sliced

¼ cup macadamia nuts, whole

1 tbsp flaxseed

1 tbsp hemp seed

1 cup water

Directions:

Add all ingredients in blender.

Blend until smooth and creamy.

Serve and enjoy.

Nutrition:

Calories per serving: 590; Carbohydrates: 17.7g; Protein: 12.3g; Fat: 57.2g; Sugar: 3.8g; Sodium: 22mg; Fiber: 10.1g

Nutty Greens Shake

Servings:  1

Ingredients:

½ cup heavy cream, liquid

1 packet Stevia, or more to taste

¼ cup pecans

¼ macadamia nuts

1 ½ cups water

1 cup Spring mix salad greens

Directions:

Add all ingredients in blender.

Blend until smooth and creamy.

Serve and enjoy.

Nutrition:

Calories per serving: 628; Carbohydrates: 12.5g; Protein: 7.0g; Fat: 65.6g; Sugar: 4.7g; Sodium: 48mg; Fiber: 6.4g

## Raspberry and Greens Shake

Preparation Time: 20 MINUTES

Servings:  1

Ingredients:

1 cup whole milk

1 packet Stevia, or more to taste

¼ cup Raspberry

1 cup water

1 tbsp macadamia oil

1 cup Spinach

Directions:

Add all ingredients in blender.

Blend until smooth and creamy.

Serve and enjoy.

Nutrition:

Calories per serving: 292; Carbohydrates: 17.43g; Protein: 8.9g; Fat: 21.9g; Sugar: 13.8g; Sodium: 136mg; Fiber: 2.7g

## Spiced Almond Shake

Preparation Time: 20 MINUTES

Servings:  1

Ingredients:

½ cup whole milk

1 tbsp cocoa powder

1 packet Stevia, or more to taste

¼ cup almonds, sliced

½ tsp cinnamon

¼ tsp allspice

¼ tsp nutmeg

1 cup water

1 tbsp almond oil

Directions:

Add all ingredients in blender.

Blend until smooth and creamy.

Serve and enjoy.

Nutrition:

Calories per serving: 347; Carbohydrates: 16.6g; Protein: 9.8g; Fat: 30.1g; Sugar: 7.3g; Sodium: 59mg; Fiber: 5.4g

## Cinnamon-Choco Coffee Milk Shake

Preparation Time: 20 Minutes

Servings:  1

Ingredients:

1 cup whole milk

1 tbsp cocoa powder

1 cup brewed coffee, chilled

½ tsp cinnamon

1 packet Stevia, or more to taste

1 tbsp coconut oil

Directions:

Add all ingredients in blender.

Blend until smooth and creamy.

Serve and enjoy.

Nutrition:

Calories per serving: 284; Carbohydrates: 16.9g; Protein: 9g; Fat: 22.3g; Sugar: 12.4g; Sodium: 111mg; Fiber: 2.3g

## Mocha Milk Shake

Preparation Time: 20 Minutes

Servings: 1

Ingredients:

1 cup whole milk

2 tbsps cocoa powder

2 packet Stevia, or more to taste

1 cup brewed coffee, chilled

1 tbsp coconut oil

Directions:

Add all ingredients in blender.

Blend until smooth and creamy.

Serve and enjoy.

Nutrition:

Calories per serving: 293; Carbohydrates: 19.9g; Protein: 10.1g; Fat: 23.1g; Sugar: 12.5g; Sodium: 112mg; Fiber: 4g

## Coconut-Mocha Shake

Preparation Time: 20 Minutes

Servings: 1

Ingredients:

3/4 cup whole milk

2 tbsps cocoa powder

1 tbsp coconut flakes, unsweetened

2 packet Stevia, or more to taste

1 cup brewed coffee, chilled

1 tbsp coconut oil

Directions:

Add all ingredients in blender.

Blend until smooth and creamy.

Serve and enjoy.

Nutrition:

Calories per serving: 280; Carbohydrates: 19.75g; Protein: 8.33g; Fat: 22.6g; Sugar: 11.4g; Sodium: 101mg; Fiber: 4.5g

## Nutritiously Green Milk Shake

Preparation Time: 20 Minutes

Servings: 1

Ingredients:

1 cup whole milk

1 packet Stevia, or more to taste

1 tbsp coconut flakes, unsweetened

1 cup water

2 cups Spring Mix Salad

1 tbsp coconut oil

Directions:

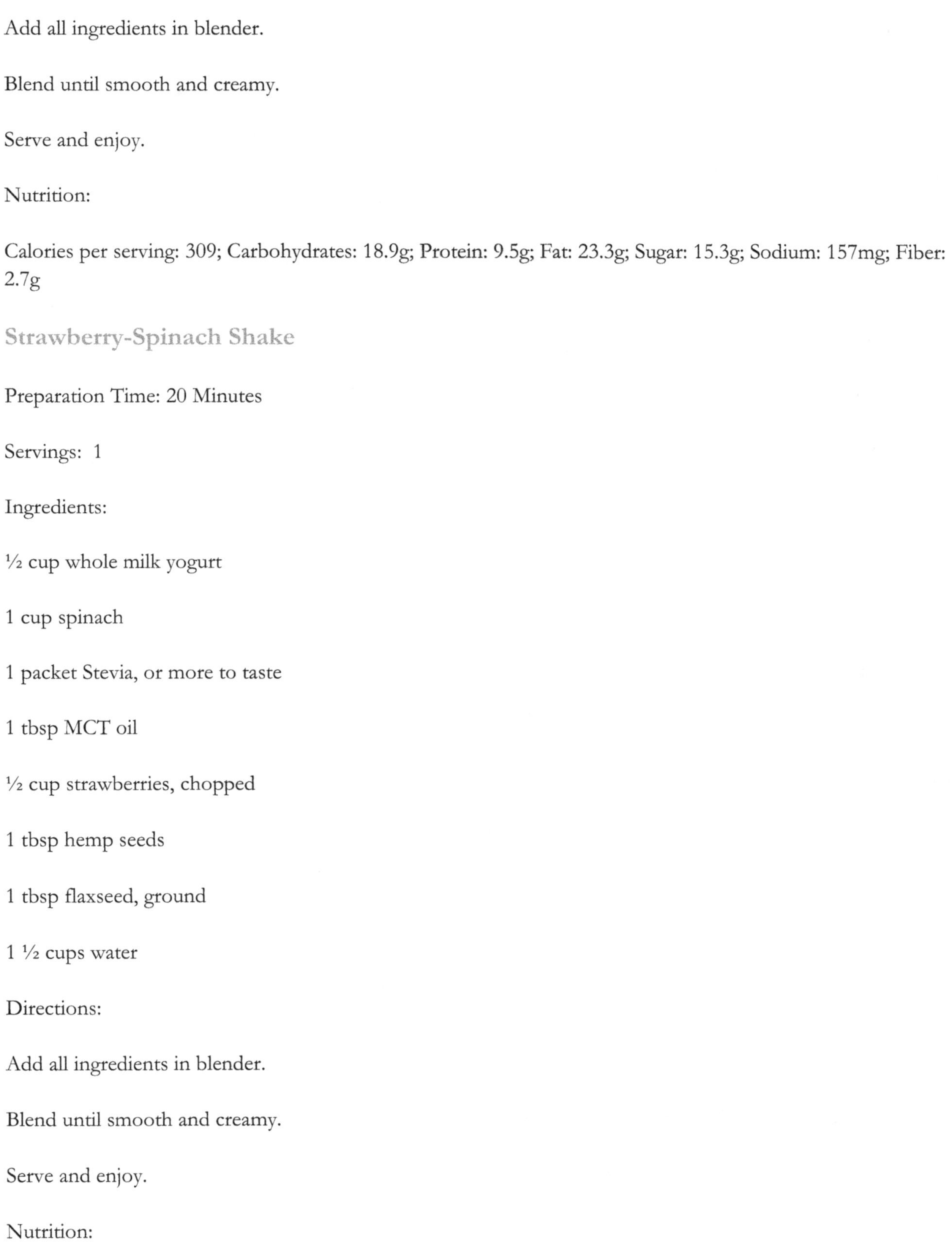

Add all ingredients in blender.

Blend until smooth and creamy.

Serve and enjoy.

Nutrition:

Calories per serving: 309; Carbohydrates: 18.9g; Protein: 9.5g; Fat: 23.3g; Sugar: 15.3g; Sodium: 157mg; Fiber: 2.7g

## Strawberry-Spinach Shake

Preparation Time: 20 Minutes

Servings:  1

Ingredients:

½ cup whole milk yogurt

1 cup spinach

1 packet Stevia, or more to taste

1 tbsp MCT oil

½ cup strawberries, chopped

1 tbsp hemp seeds

1 tbsp flaxseed, ground

1 ½ cups water

Directions:

Add all ingredients in blender.

Blend until smooth and creamy.

Serve and enjoy.

Nutrition:

Calories per serving: 334; Carbohydrates: 18.9g; Protein: 9.4g; Fat: 26.7g; Sugar: 10.3g; Sodium: 90mg; Fiber: 5.9g

## Lemon-Mint Creamy Green Smoothie

Preparation Time: 20 Minutes

Servings:  1

Ingredients:

½ cup whole milk yogurt

1 cup Spring mix salad greens, packed

1 packet Stevia, or more to taste

1 tbsp MCT oil

1 tsp lemon juice, fresh

2 peppermint leaves

1 tbsp chia seeds

1 tbsp flaxseed, ground

1 ½ cups water

Directions:

Add all ingredients in blender.

Blend until smooth and creamy.

Serve and enjoy.

Nutrition:

Calories per serving: 326; Carbohydrates: 17.1g; Protein: 9.4g; Fat: 26.3g; Sugar: 6.1g; Sodium: 91mg; Fiber: 8.4g

## 5-Lettuce Mix Green Shake

Preparation Time: 20 Minutes

Servings:  1

Ingredients:

¾ cup whole milk yogurt

2 cups 5-lettuce mix salad greens

1 packet Stevia, or more to taste

1 tbsp MCT oil

1 tbsp chia seeds

1 ½ cups water

Directions:

Add all ingredients in blender.

Blend until smooth and creamy.

Serve and enjoy.

Nutrition:

Calories per serving: 320; Carbohydrates: 19.1g; Protein: 10.4g; Fat: 24.2g; Sugar: 9.6g; Sodium: 126mg; Fiber: 7.1g

## Basil and Pine Nuts Shake

Preparation Time: 20 Minutes

Servings:  1

Ingredients:

½ cup whole milk yogurt

1 cup spring mix salad greens

1 packet Stevia, or more to taste

1 tbsp olive oil

2 tbsps pine nuts, chopped

2 tbsps walnuts, chopped

10 basil leaves

1 tbsp hemp seeds

1 ½ cups water

Directions:

Add all ingredients in blender.

Blend until smooth and creamy.

Serve and enjoy.

Nutrition:

Calories per serving: 465; Carbohydrates: 14.6g; Protein: 11.6g; Fat: 43.2g; Sugar: 7.4g; Sodium: 81mg; Fiber: 3.5g

## Rosemary-Lemon Garden Greens Smoothie

Preparation Time: 20 Minutes

Servings:  1

Ingredients:

½ cup whole milk yogurt

1 cup Garden greens

1 packet Stevia, or more to taste

1 tbsp olive oil

1 stalk fresh rosemary

1 tbsp lemon juice, fresh

1 tbsp pepitas

1 tbsp flaxseed, ground

1 ½ cups water

Directions:

Add all ingredients in blender.

Blend until smooth and creamy.

Serve and enjoy.

Nutrition:

Calories per serving: 312; Carbohydrates: 14.7g; Protein: 9.7g; Fat: 25.9g; Sugar: 8.6g; Sodium: 75mg; Fiber: 4g

## Lemon-Cilantro Greens Shake

Preparation Time: 20 Minutes

Servings:  1

Ingredients:

½ cup whole milk yogurt

1 cup baby kale greens

1 packet Stevia, or more to taste

1 tbsp avocado oil

1 tbsp lemon juice, fresh

1 tsp cilantro, chopped

¼ avocado fruit

1 tbsp flaxseed, ground

1 ½ cups water

Directions:

Add all ingredients in blender.

Blend until smooth and creamy.

Serve and enjoy.

Nutrition:

Calories per serving: 345; Carbohydrates: 16.4g; Protein: 7.9g; Fat: 29.9g; Sugar: 6.9g; Sodium: 76mg; Fiber: 6.8g

## Blackberry-Chocolate Shake

Preparation Time: 20 Minutes

Servings:  1

Ingredients:

½ cup whole milk yogurt

¼ cup blackberries

1 packet Stevia, or more to taste

1 tbsp MCT oil

1 tbsp Dutch-processed cocoa powder

2 tbsps Macadamia nuts, chopped

1 ½ cups water

Directions:

Add all ingredients in blender.

Blend until smooth and creamy.

Serve and enjoy.

Nutrition:

Calories per serving: 463; Carbohydrates: 17.9g; Protein: 8.5g; Fat: 43.9g; Sugar: 9.1g; Sodium: 67mg; Fiber: 6.8g

## Strawberry-Coconut Shake

Preparation Time: 20 Min

Servings:  1

Ingredients:

½ cup whole milk yogurt

1 packet Stevia, or more to taste

1 tbsp MCT oil

¼ cup strawberries, chopped

1 tbsp coconut flakes, unsweetened

1 tbsp hemp seeds

1 ½ cups water

Directions:

Add all ingredients in blender.

Blend until smooth and creamy.

Serve and enjoy.

Nutrition:

Calories per serving: 282; Carbohydrates: 14.0g; Protein: 6.5g; Fat: 23.7g; Sugar: 9.6g; Sodium: 80mg; Fiber: 2g

## Coconut-Melon Yogurt Shake

Preparation Time: 20 Min

Servings:  1

Ingredients:

¼ cup whole milk yogurt

1 packet Stevia, or more to taste

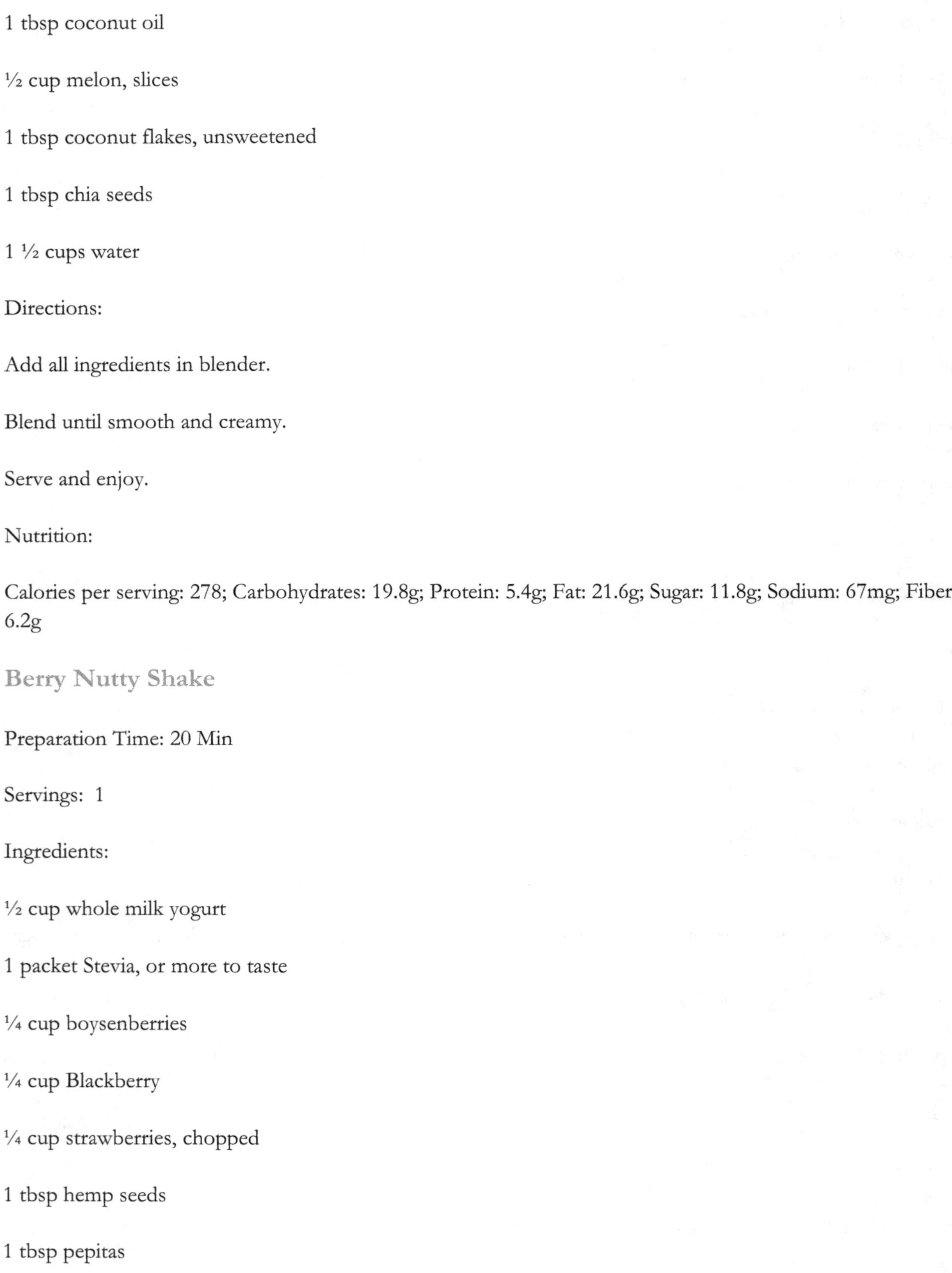

1 tbsp coconut oil

½ cup melon, slices

1 tbsp coconut flakes, unsweetened

1 tbsp chia seeds

1 ½ cups water

Directions:

Add all ingredients in blender.

Blend until smooth and creamy.

Serve and enjoy.

Nutrition:

Calories per serving: 278; Carbohydrates: 19.8g; Protein: 5.4g; Fat: 21.6g; Sugar: 11.8g; Sodium: 67mg; Fiber: 6.2g

## Berry Nutty Shake

Preparation Time: 20 Min

Servings:  1

Ingredients:

½ cup whole milk yogurt

1 packet Stevia, or more to taste

¼ cup boysenberries

¼ cup Blackberry

¼ cup strawberries, chopped

1 tbsp hemp seeds

1 tbsp pepitas

1 tbsp chia seeds

1 ½ cups water

Directions:

Add all ingredients in blender.

Blend until smooth and creamy.

Serve and enjoy.

Nutrition:

Calories per serving: 283; Carbohydrates: 26.2g; Protein: 11.8g; Fat: 16.9g; Sugar: 12.1g; Sodium: 69mg; Fiber: 10.6g

## Berry Overload Shake

Preparation Time: 20 Min

Servings:  1

Ingredients:

½ cup whole milk yogurt

1 packet Stevia, or more to taste

¼ cup blueberries

¼ cup boysenberries

¼ cup Blackberry

¼ cup strawberries, chopped

1 tbsp avocado oil

1 ½ cups water

Directions:

Add all ingredients in blender.

Blend until smooth and creamy.

Serve and enjoy.

Nutrition:

Calories per serving: 263; Carbohydrates: 22.3g; Protein: 5.6g; Fat: 18.5g; Sugar: 15.2g; Sodium: 65mg; Fiber: 5.3g

## Berry-Choco Goodness Shake

Preparation Time: 20 Min

Servings:  1

Ingredients:

½ cup whole milk yogurt

1 packet Stevia, or more to taste

¼ cup raspberries

¼ cup Blackberry

¼ cup strawberries, chopped

1 tbsp cocoa powder

1 tbsp avocado oil

1 ½ cups water

Directions:

Add all ingredients in blender.

Blend until smooth and creamy.

Serve and enjoy.

Nutrition:

Calories per serving: 255; Carbohydrates: 20.2g; Protein: 6.4g; Fat: 19.2g; Sugar: 11.0g; Sodium: 66mg; Fiber: 6.3g

## Lemony-Avocado Cilantro Shake

Preparation Time: 20 Min

Servings:  1

Ingredients:

½ cup whole milk yogurt

1 packet Stevia, or more to taste

1 whole avocado

1 tbsp chopped cilantro

1 ½ cups water

Directions:

Add all ingredients in blender.

Blend until smooth and creamy.

Serve and enjoy.

Nutrition:

Calories per serving: 397; Carbohydrates: 23.4g; Protein: 8.3g; Fat: 33.4g; Sugar: 7.0g; Sodium: 78mg; Fiber: 13.5g

## Strawberry-Chocolate Yogurt Shake

Preparation Time: 20 Min

Servings:  1

Ingredients:

½ cup whole milk yogurt

1 packet Stevia, or more to taste

½ cup strawberries, chopped

1 tbsp cocoa powder

1 tbsp coconut oil

1 tbsp pepitas

1 ½ cups water

Directions:

Add all ingredients in blender.

Blend until smooth and creamy.

Serve and enjoy.

Nutrition:

Calories per serving: 269; Carbohydrates: 16.5g; Protein: g; Fat: 7.9g; Sugar: 9.4g; Sodium: 67mg; Fiber: 3.5g

## Blueberry and Greens Smoothie

Preparation Time: 20 Min

Servings:  1

Ingredients:

½ cup coconut milk

1 ½ cups water

½ cup blueberries

2 packets Stevia, or as needed

1 cup arugula

1 tbsp hemp seeds

Directions:

Add all ingredients in blender.

Blend until smooth and creamy.

Serve and enjoy.

Nutrition:

Calories per serving: 321; Carbohydrates: 18.4g; Protein: 5.2g; Fat: 29.0g; Sugar: 8.0g; Sodium: 29mg; Fiber: 2.9g

## Avocado and Greens Smoothie

Preparation Time: 20 Min

Servings:  1

Ingredients:

½ cup coconut milk

1 ½ cups water

½ Avocado fruit

2 packets Stevia, or as needed

1 cup Spring mix greens

1 tbsp avocado oil

Directions:

Add all ingredients in blender.

Blend until smooth and creamy.

Serve and enjoy.

Nutrition:

Calories per serving: 439; Carbohydrates: 16.1g; Protein: 6.5g; Fat: 43.4g; Sugar: 1.0g; Sodium: 37mg; Fiber: 7.7g

# Chapter 3.      Soup Recipes

## Cauliflower Soup

Preparation Time:  10 minutes

Cooking Time: 4 hours 5 minutes

Servings: 04

Ingredients:

2 tablespoons olive oil

1½ cups sweet white onion, chopped

2 large cloves of garlic, chopped

1 head cauliflower, cut into florets

1 cup coconut milk

1 cup filtered water

1 teaspoon vegetable stock paste

2 tablespoons nutritional yeast

Dash of olive oil

Fresh cracked pepper

Parsley, to serve

Directions:

Add olive oil and onion to a slow cooker.

Sauté for 5 minutes then add the rest of the ingredients.

Put on the slow cooker's lid and cook for 4 hours on low heat.

Once done, blend the soup with a hand blender.

Garnish with parsley, and cracked pepper

Serve.

Nutrition:

Calories 119

Total Fat 14 g

Saturated Fat 2 g

Cholesterol 65 mg

Sodium 269 mg

Total Carbs 19 g

Fiber 4 g

Sugar 6 g

Protein 5g

## Greek Lentil Soup

Preparation Time:  10 minutes

Cooking Time: 6 hours 2 minutes

Servings: 04

Ingredients:

Soup:

1 cup lentils

1 medium sweet onion, chopped

2 large carrots, chopped

2 sticks of celery, chopped

4 cups veggie broth

Olive oil to sauté

4 tablespoons tomato sauce

3 cloves garlic

3 bay leaves

Salt, to taste

Black pepper, to taste

Dried oregano, to taste

Toppings:

Vinegar

Lemon juice

Hot sauce

Directions:

In a slow cooker, add olive oil and onion.

Sauté for 2 minutes then add the rest of the soup ingredients.

Put on the slow cooker's lid and cook for 6 hours on low heat.

Serve warm with the vinegar, lemon juice, and hot sauce.

Nutrition:

Calories 231

Total Fat 20.1 g

Saturated Fat 2.4 g

Cholesterol 110 mg

Sodium 941 mg

Total Carbs 20.1 g

Fiber 0.9 g

Sugar 1.4 g

Protein 4.6 g

## Broccoli White Bean Soup

Preparation Time:  10 minutes

Cooking Time: 4 hrs. 32 minutes

Servings: 04

Ingredients:

1 large bunch broccoli

3 cloves garlic

1 medium white potato

¼ cup carrot, chopped

2 cups almond milk

1½ cups white beans, cooked

1 white onion, chopped

¾ teaspoon black pepper

¼ teaspoon salt

½ teaspoon smoky paprika

⅓ cup nutritional yeast

1 bay leaf

1 cup cooked pasta

Directions:

In a slow cooker, add olive oil and onion.

Sauté for 2 minutes then toss in the rest of the ingredients except pasta and beans.

Put on the slow cooker's lid and cook for 4 hours on low heat.

Once done, add pasta and beans to the soup and mix gently.

Cover the soup and remove it from the heat then leave it for another 30 minutes.

Serve warm.

Nutrition:

Calories 361

Total Fat 16.3 g

Saturated Fat 4.9 g

Cholesterol 114 mg

Sodium 515 mg

Total Carbs 29.3 g

Fiber 0.1 g

Sugar 18.2 g

Protein 3.3 g

## African Lentil Soup

Preparation Time:  10 minutes

Cooking Time: 20 minutes

Servings: 4

Ingredients:

1 teaspoon oil

½ medium onion, chopped

2 juicy tomatoes, chopped

1½ teaspoons ground cumin

4 garlic cloves, chopped

1-inch piece of ginger, chopped

1 tablespoon Sambal Oelek

¼ teaspoon black pepper

1 teaspoon Harissa Spice Blend

¼ cup nut butter

2 tablespoons peanuts

½ cup red lentils

2 teaspoons ground coriander

2½ cups vegetable stock

1 tablespoon tomato paste

¾ teaspoon salt

1 teaspoon lemon juice

½ cup packed baby spinach

Directions:

In a slow cooker, add olive oil and onion.

Sauté for 5 minutes then toss in rest of the ingredients except peanuts.

Put on the slow cooker's lid and cook for 5 hours on low heat.

Once done, garnish with peanuts.

Serve.

Nutrition:

Calories 205

Total Fat 22.7 g

Saturated Fat 6.1 g

Cholesterol 4 mg

Sodium 227 mg

Total Carbs 26.1 g

Fiber 1.4 g

Sugar 0.9 g

Protein 5.2 g

Preparation Time:  10 minutes

Cooking Time: 20 minutes

Servings: 04

Ingredients:

1 (15 ounce) can artichoke hearts

½ bunch kale, chopped

2 cups vegetable broth

1 tablespoon dried basil

1 tablespoon dried oregano

1 teaspoon salt

½ teaspoon red pepper flakes

Black pepper, to taste

2 (14 ounce) cans roasted tomatoes, diced

1 (15 ounce) can white beans, drained

Directions:

Add all ingredients to a saucepan.

Put on the saucepan's lid and cook for 20 minutes on a simmer.

Serve warm.

Nutrition:

Calories 201

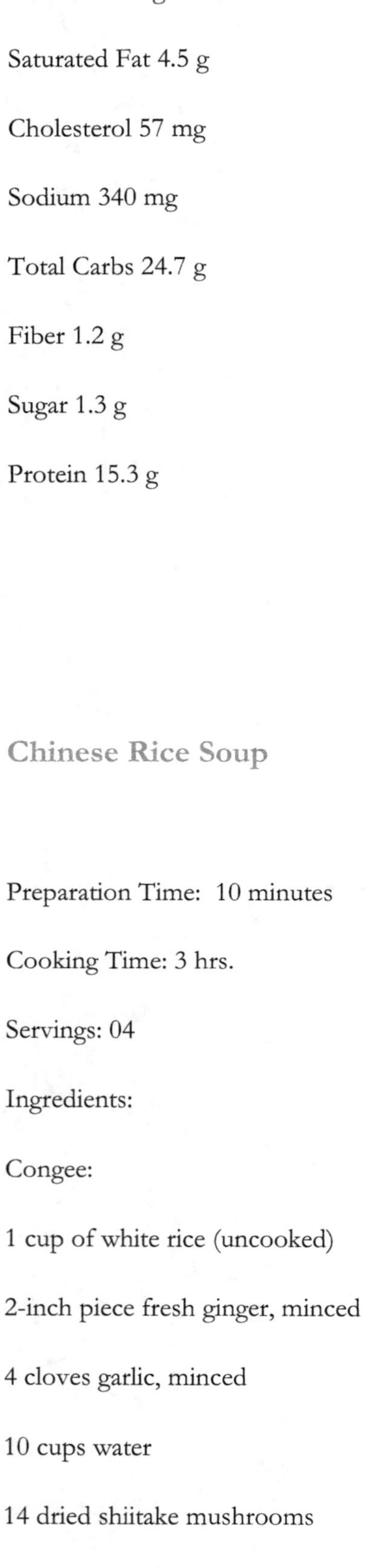

Total Fat 8.9 g

Saturated Fat 4.5 g

Cholesterol 57 mg

Sodium 340 mg

Total Carbs 24.7 g

Fiber 1.2 g

Sugar 1.3 g

Protein 15.3 g

## Chinese Rice Soup

Preparation Time:  10 minutes

Cooking Time: 3 hrs.

Servings: 04

Ingredients:

Congee:

1 cup of white rice (uncooked)

2-inch piece fresh ginger, minced

4 cloves garlic, minced

10 cups water

14 dried shiitake mushrooms

Toppings:

Green onions

Cilantro

Sesame seeds

Hot sauce

Toasted sesame oil

Soy sauce

Peanuts

Chili oil

Shelled edamame

Directions:

Add all the ingredients to a slow cooker.

Put on the slow cooker's lid and cook for 3 hours on low heat.

Once done, garnish with desired toppings.

Serve warm.

Nutrition:

Calories 210.6

Total Fat 10.91g

Saturated Fat 7.4g

Sodium 875 mg

Potassium 604 mg

Carbohydrates 25.6g

Fiber 4.3g

Sugar 7.9g

Protein 2.1g

## Black-eyed Pea Soup with Greens

Preparation Time:  10 minutes

Cooking Time: 5 hrs.

Servings: 04

Ingredients:

½ cup black eyed peas

½ cup brown lentils

1 teaspoon oil

½ teaspoon cumin seeds

½ cup onions, chopped

5 cloves garlic, chopped

1-inch piece of ginger chopped

1 teaspoon ground coriander

½ teaspoon ground cumin

½ teaspoon turmeric

¼ teaspoon black pepper

½ teaspoon cayenne powder

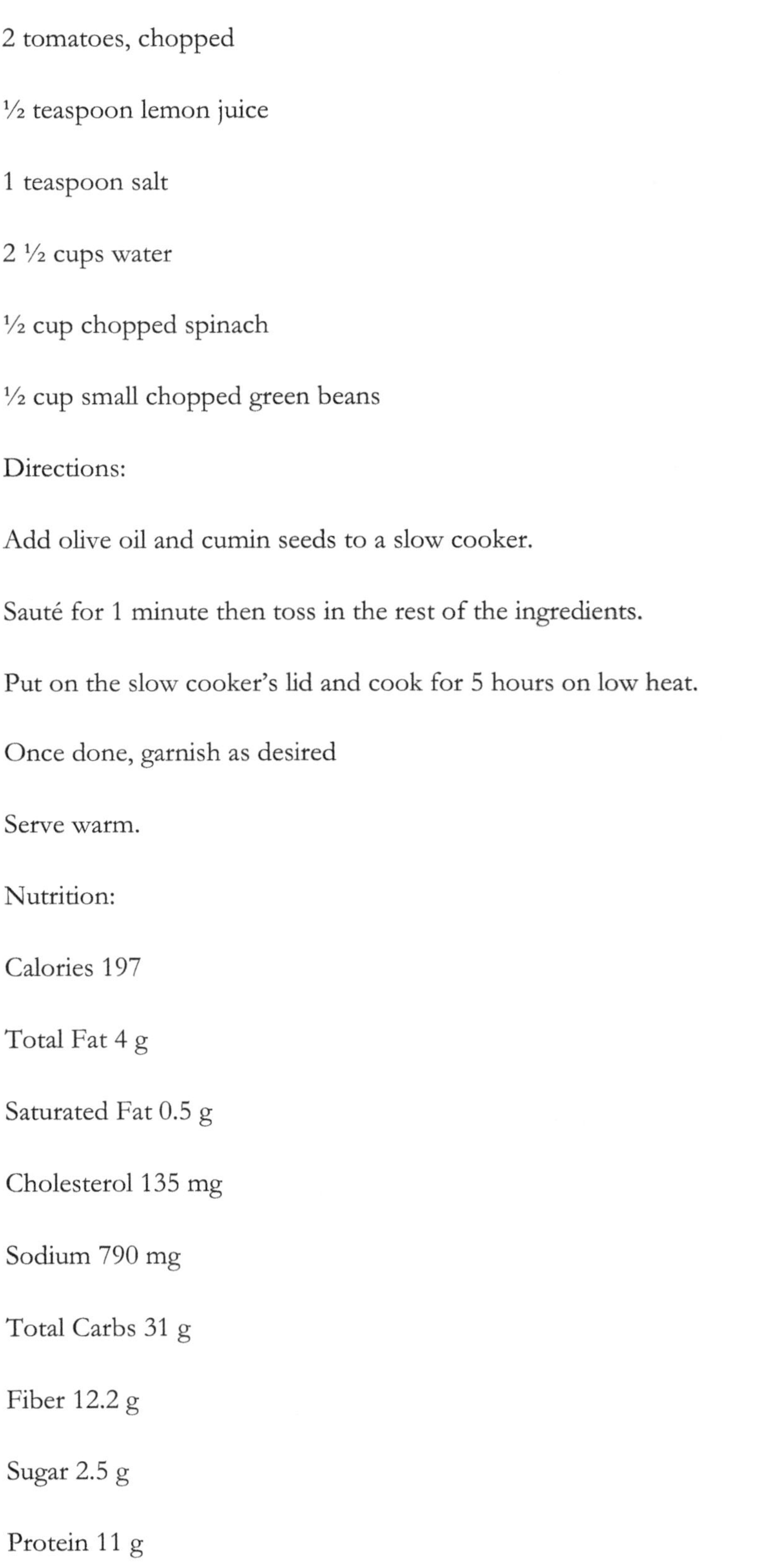

2 tomatoes, chopped

½ teaspoon lemon juice

1 teaspoon salt

2 ½ cups water

½ cup chopped spinach

½ cup small chopped green beans

Directions:

Add olive oil and cumin seeds to a slow cooker.

Sauté for 1 minute then toss in the rest of the ingredients.

Put on the slow cooker's lid and cook for 5 hours on low heat.

Once done, garnish as desired

Serve warm.

Nutrition:

Calories 197

Total Fat 4 g

Saturated Fat 0.5 g

Cholesterol 135 mg

Sodium 790 mg

Total Carbs 31 g

Fiber 12.2 g

Sugar 2.5 g

Protein 11 g

# Beanless Garden Soup

Preparation Time:  10 minutes

Cooking Time: 4 hrs. 5 minutes

Servings: 04

Ingredients:

1 medium onion, diced

2 cloves garlic, minced

1 green bell pepper, diced

1 red bell pepper, diced

2 carrots, peeled and diced

1 medium zucchini, diced

1 small eggplant, diced

1 hot banana pepper, seeded and minced

1 jalapeño pepper, seeded and minced

1 can (28 ounce) diced tomatoes

3 cups vegetable broth

1½ tablespoon chili powder

2 teaspoons smoked paprika

1 tablespoon cumin

2 tablespoons fresh oregano, chopped

2 tablespoons fresh cilantro, chopped

Salt and black pepper to taste

A few dashes of liquid smoke

Directions:

In a slow cooker, add olive oil and onion.

Sauté for 5 minutes then toss in the rest of the ingredients.

Put on the slow cooker's lid and cook for 4 hours on low heat.

Once done mix well.

Serve warm.

Nutrition:

Calories 305

Total Fat 11.8 g

Saturated Fat 2.2 g

Cholesterol 56 mg

Sodium 321 mg

Total Carbs 34.6 g

Fibers 0.4 g

Sugar 2 g

Protein 7 g

# Black-eyed Pea Soup with Olive Pesto

Preparation Time:  10 minutes

Cooking Time: 3 hrs. 5 minutes

Servings: 04

Ingredients:

Soup:

1 leek, trimmed

1 tablespoon olive oil

1 clove garlic, chopped

1 small carrot, chopped

1 stem fresh thyme, chopped

1 (15 ounce) can black-eyed peas, drained and rinsed

2½ cups vegetable broth

½ teaspoon salt

¼ teaspoon black pepper

Pesto:

1¼ cups pitted green olives

¼ cup parsley leaves

1 clove garlic

1 teaspoon capers, drained

1 tablespoon olive oil

Directions:

In a slow cooker, add olive oil, carrot, leek, and garlic.

Sauté for 5 minutes then toss in the rest of the soup ingredients.

Put on the slow cooker's lid and cook for 3 hours on low heat.

Meanwhile, blend the pesto ingredients in a blender until smooth.

Blend the soup in the slow cooker with a hand mixer.

Top with prepared pesto.

Serve warm.

Nutrition:

Calories 72

Total Fat 15.4 g

Saturated Fat 4.2 g

Cholesterol 168 mg

Sodium 203 mg

Total Carbs 28.5 g

Sugar 1.1 g

Fiber 4 g

Protein 7.9 g

Spinach Soup with Basil

Preparation Time:  10 minutes

Cooking Time: 5hrs. 5 minutes

Servings: 06

Ingredients:

8 ounces potatoes, diced

1 medium onion, chopped

1 large clove of garlic, chopped

1 teaspoon powdered mustard

3 cups water

¼ teaspoon salt

Ground cayenne pepper

½ cup packed fresh dill

10 ounces frozen spinach

Directions:

In a low cooker, add olive oil and onion.

Sauté for 5 minutes then toss in rest of the soup ingredients.

Put on the slow cooker's lid and cook for 5 hours on low heat.

Once done, puree the soup with a hand blender.

Serve warm.

Nutrition:

Calories 162

Total Fat 4 g

Saturated Fat 1.9 g

Cholesterol 25 mg

Sodium 101 mg

Total Carbs 17.8 g

Sugar 2.1 g

Fiber 6 g

Protein 4 g

## Red Lentil Salsa Soup

Preparation Time:  10 minutes

Cooking Time: 17 minutes

Preparation Time: 27 minutes

Servings: 06

Ingredients:

1¼ cups red lentils, rinsed

4 cups of water

½ cup diced red bell pepper

1¼ cups red salsa

1 tablespoon chili powder

1 tablespoon dried oregano

1 teaspoon smoked paprika

¼ teaspoon black pepper

¾ cup frozen sweet corn

Salt to taste

2 tablespoons lime juice

Directions:

In a saucepan, add all the ingredients except the corn.

Put on saucepan's lid and cook for 15 minutes at a simmer.

Stir in corn and cook for another 2 minutes.

Serve.

Nutrition:

Calories 119

Total Fat 14 g

Saturated Fat 2 g

Cholesterol 65 mg

Sodium 269 mg

Total Carbs 19 g

Fiber 4 g

Sugar 6 g

Protein 5g

# Caldo Verde a la Mushrooms

Preparation Time:  10 minutes

Cooking Time: 5 hrs. 5 minutes

Servings: 08

Ingredients:

¼ cup olive oil

10 ounces button mushrooms, cleaned, and sliced

1½ teaspoons smoked paprika

1 pinch ground cayenne pepper

1 teaspoon salt

1 large onion, diced

2 cloves garlic, minced

2 pounds russet potatoes, peeled and diced

7 cups vegetable broth

8 ounces kale, sliced

½ teaspoon black pepper

Directions:

In a pan, heat cooking oil and sauté mushrooms for 12 minutes.

Season the mushrooms with salt, cayenne pepper, and paprika.

Add olive oil and onion to a slow cooker.

Sauté for 5 minutes then toss in rest of the soup ingredients.

Put on the slow cooker's lid and cook for 5 hours on low heat.

Once done, puree the soup with a hand blender.

Stir in sautéed mushrooms.

Serve.

Nutrition:

Calories 231

Total Fat 20.1 g

Saturated Fat 2.4 g

Cholesterol 110 mg

Sodium 941 mg

Total Carbs 20.1 g

Fiber 0.9 g

Sugar 1.4 g

Protein 4.6 g

## Shiitake Mushroom Split Pea Soup

Preparation Time:  10 minutes

Cooking Time: 6 hours

Preparation Time: 6 hours 10 minutes

Servings: 12

Ingredients:

1 cup dried, green split peas

2 cups celery, chopped

2 cups sliced carrots

1½ cups cauliflower, chopped

2 ounces dried shiitake mushrooms, chopped

9 ounces frozen artichoke hearts

11 cups water

1 teaspoon garlic powder

1½ teaspoon onion powder

½ teaspoon black pepper

1 tablespoon parsley

½ teaspoon ginger

½ teaspoon ground mustard seed

½ tablespoon brown rice vinegar

Directions:

Add all the ingredients to a slow cooker.

Put on the slow cooker's lid and cook for 6 hours on low heat.

Once done, garnish as desired.

Serve warm.

Nutrition:

Calories 361

Total Fat 16.3 g

Saturated Fat 4.9 g

Cholesterol 114 mg

Sodium 515 mg

Total Carbs 29.3 g

Fiber 0.1 g

Sugar 18.2 g

Protein 3.3 g

## Velvety Vegetable Soup

Preparation Time:  10 minutes

Cooking Time: 2hrs 2 minutes

Servings: 4

Ingredients:

½ sweet onion, chopped

4 garlic cloves, chopped

1 small head broccoli, chopped

2 stalks celery, chopped

1 cup green peas

3 green onions, chopped

2¾ cups vegetable broth

4 cups leafy greens

1 (15 ounce) can of cannellini beans

Juice from 1 lemon

2 tablespoons fresh dill, chopped

5 fresh mint leaves

1 teaspoon salt

½ cup coconut milk

Fresh herbs and peas, to garnish

Directions:

In a slow cooker, add olive oil and onion.

Sauté for 2 minutes then toss in the rest of the soup ingredients.

Put on the slow cooker's lid and cook for 2 hours on low heat.

Once done, blend the soup with a hand blender.

Garnish with fresh herbs and peas.

Serve warm.

Nutrition:

Calories 205

Total Fat 22.7 g

Saturated Fat 6.1 g

Cholesterol 4 mg

Sodium 227 mg

Total Carbs 26.1 g

Fiber 1.4 g

Sugar 0.9 g

Protein 5.2 g

## Sweet Potato and Peanut Soup

Preparation Time:  10 minutes

Cooking Time: 4 hrs. 5 minutes

Servings: 06

Ingredients:

1 tablespoon water

6 cups sweet potatoes, peeled and chopped

2 cups onions, chopped

1 cup celery, chopped

4 large cloves garlic, chopped

1 teaspoon salt

2 teaspoons cumin seeds

3½ teaspoons ground coriander

1 teaspoon paprika

½ teaspoon crushed red pepper flakes

2 cups vegetable stock

3 cups water

4 tablespoons fresh ginger, grated

2 tablespoons natural peanut butter

2 cups cooked chickpeas

4 tablespoons lime juice

Fresh cilantro, chopped

Chopped peanuts, to garnish

Directions:

In a slow cooker, add olive oil and onion.

Sauté for 5 minutes then toss in the rest of the soup ingredients except chickpeas.

Put on the slow cooker's lid and cook for 4 hours on low heat.

Once done, blend the soup with a hand blender.

Stir in chickpeas and garnish with cilantro and peanuts.

Serve warm.

Nutrition:

Calories 201

Total Fat 8.9 g

Saturated Fat 4.5 g

Cholesterol 57 mg

Sodium 340 mg

Total Carbs 24.7 g

Fiber 1.2 g

Sugar 1.3 g

Protein 15.3 g

# Chapter 4.  Stir-Fried, Grilled, & Hashed Vegetables

## Crusty Grilled Corn

Preparation Time: 10 minutes

Cooking Time: 15 minutes

Servings: 4

Ingredients

2 corn cobs

1/3 cup Vegenaise

1 small handful cilantro

½ cup breadcrumbs

1 teaspoon lemon juice

Directions

Preheat the gas grill on high heat.

Add corn grill to the grill and continue grilling until it turns golden-brown on all sides.

Mix the Vegenaise, cilantro, breadcrumbs, and lemon juice in a bowl.

Add grilled corn cobs to the crumbs mixture.

Toss well then serve.

Nutritional Values

Calories: 372

Total Fat: 11.1 g

Saturated Fat: 5.8 g

Cholesterol: 610 mg

Sodium: 749 mg

Total Carbs: 16.9 g

Fiber: 0.2 g

Sugar: 0.2 g

Protein: 13.5 g

## Grilled Carrots with Chickpea Salad

Preparation Time: 10 minutes

Cooking Time: 10 minutes

Servings: 8

Ingredients

Carrots

8 large carrots

1 tablespoon oil

1 ½ teaspoon salt

1 teaspoon dried oregano

1 teaspoon dried thyme

2 teaspoon paprika powder

1 ½ tablespoon soy sauce

½ cup of water

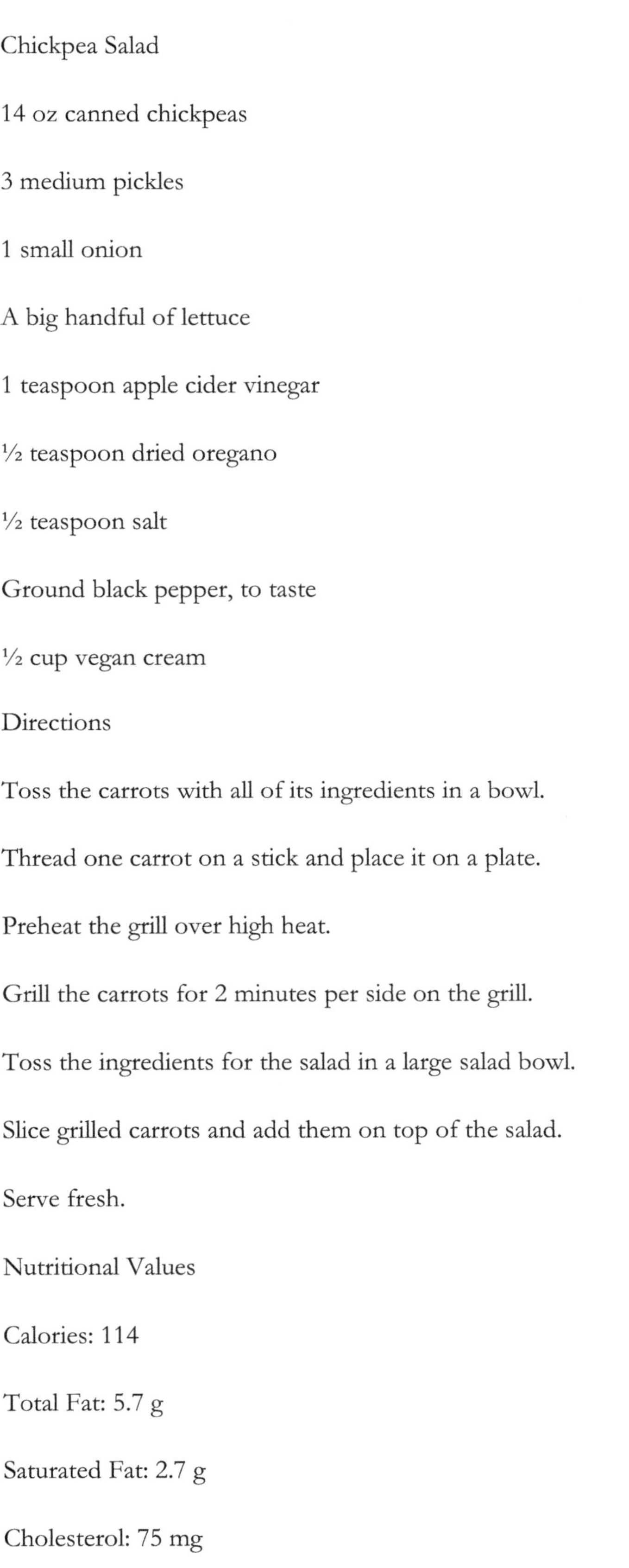

Chickpea Salad

14 oz canned chickpeas

3 medium pickles

1 small onion

A big handful of lettuce

1 teaspoon apple cider vinegar

½ teaspoon dried oregano

½ teaspoon salt

Ground black pepper, to taste

½ cup vegan cream

Directions

Toss the carrots with all of its ingredients in a bowl.

Thread one carrot on a stick and place it on a plate.

Preheat the grill over high heat.

Grill the carrots for 2 minutes per side on the grill.

Toss the ingredients for the salad in a large salad bowl.

Slice grilled carrots and add them on top of the salad.

Serve fresh.

Nutritional Values

Calories: 114

Total Fat: 5.7 g

Saturated Fat: 2.7 g

Cholesterol: 75 mg

Sodium: 94 mg

Total Carbs: 31.4 g

Fiber: 0.6 g

Sugar: 15 g

Protein: 4.1 g

## Grilled Avocado Guacamole

Preparation Time: 10 minutes

Cooking Time: 20 minutes

Servings: 4

Ingredients

½ teaspoon olive oil

1 lime, halved

½ onion, halved

1 serrano chile, halved, stemmed, and seeded

3 Haas avocados, skin on

2–3 tablespoons fresh cilantro, chopped

½ teaspoon smoked salt

Directions

Preheat the grill over medium heat.

Brush the grilling grates with olive oil and place chile, onion, and lime on it.

Grill the onion for 10 minutes, chile for 5 minutes, and lime for 2 minutes.

Transfer the veggies to a large bowl.

Now cut the avocados in half and grill them for 5 minutes.

Mash the flesh of the grilled avocado in a bowl.

Chop the other grilled veggies and add them to the avocado mash.

Stir in remaining ingredients and mix well.

Serve.

Nutritional Values

Calories: 249

Total Fat: 11.9 g

Saturated Fat: 1.7 g

Cholesterol: 78 mg

Sodium: 79 mg

Total Carbs: 41.8 g

Fiber: 1.1 g

Sugar: 0.3 g

Protein: 1 g

Grilled Fajitas with Jalapeño Sauce

Preparation Time: 10 minutes

Cooking Time: 25 minutes

Servings: 4

Ingredients

Marinade

¼ cup olive oil

¼ cup lime juice

2 garlic cloves, minced

1 teaspoon chili powder

1 teaspoon ground cumin

1 teaspoon dried oregano

½ teaspoon salt

½ teaspoon black pepper

Jalapeño Sauce

6 jalapeno peppers stemmed, halved, and seeded

1–2 teaspoons olive oil

1 cup raw cashews, soaked and drained

½ cup almond milk

¼ cup water

¼ cup lime juice

2 teaspoons agaves

½ cup fresh cilantro

Salt, to taste

Grilled Vegetables

½ lb asparagus spears, trimmed

2 large portobello mushrooms, sliced

1 large zucchini, sliced

1 red bell pepper, sliced

1 red onion, sliced

Directions

Dump all the ingredients for the marinade in a large bowl.

Toss in all the veggies and mix well to marinate for 1 hour.

Meanwhile, prepare the sauce and brush the jalapenos with oil.

Grill the jalapenos for 5 minutes per side until slightly charred.

Blend the grilled jalapenos with other ingredients for the sauce in a blender.

Transfer this sauce to a separate bowl and keep it aside.

Now grill the marinated veggies in the grill until soft and slightly charred on all sides.

Pour the prepared sauce over the grilled veggies.

Serve.

Nutritional Values

Calories: 213

Total Fat: 14 g

Saturated Fat: 8 g

Cholesterol: 81 mg

Sodium: 162 mg

Total Carbs: 53 g

Fiber: 0.7 g

Sugar: 19 g

Protein: 12 g

## Grilled Ratatouille Kebabs

Preparation Time: 10 minutes

Cooking Time: 20 minutes

Servings: 6

Ingredients

3 tablespoons soy sauce

3 tablespoons balsamic vinegar

1 teaspoon dried thyme leaves

2 tablespoons extra virgin olive oil

Veggies

1 zucchini, diced

½ red onion, diced

½ red capsicum, diced

2 tomatoes, diced

1 small eggplant, diced

8 button mushrooms, diced

Directions

Toss the veggies with soy sauce, olive oil, thyme, and balsamic vinegar in a large bowl.

Thread the veggies alternately on the wooden skewers and reserve the remaining marinade.

Marinate these skewers for 1 hour in the refrigerator.

Preheat the grill over medium heat.

Grill the marinated skewers for 5 minutes per side while basting with the reserved marinade.

Serve fresh.

Nutritional Values

Calories: 379

Total Fat: 29.7 g

Saturated Fat: 18.6 g

Cholesterol: 141 mg

Sodium: 193 mg

Total Carbs: 23.7 g

Fiber: 0.9 g

Sugar: 1.3 g

Protein: 5.2 g

# Grilled Plantain Chips

Preparation Time: 10 minutes

Cooking Time: 14 minutes

Servings: 4

Ingredients

1 green plantain, peeled and sliced

½ teaspoon smoked paprika

¼ teaspoon cumin

Directions

Preheat the grill over medium heat.

Grease an aluminum sheet with cooking spray.

Spread the plantains in the aluminum sheet and drizzle smoked paprika and cumin on top.

Place the foil sheet with plantain slices on the grill.

Close the grill with its cover and cook for 7 minutes.

Flip the plantain slices using a tong.

Cover again and cook for 7 minutes.

Serve.

Nutritional Values

Calories: 268

Total Fat: 6 g

Saturated Fat: 1.2 g

Cholesterol: 351 mg

Sodium: 103 mg

Total Carbs: 12.8 g

Fiber: 9.2 g

Sugar: 2.9 g

Protein: 7.2 g

## Cilantro Lime Corn

Preparation Time: 10 minutes

Cooking Time: 15 minutes

Servings: 8

Ingredients

Sauce

½ cup raw cashews

½ cup water

¼ cup nutritional yeast

¼ cup lime juice

1 small handful of cilantro

1 tablespoon Dijon mustard

1 garlic clove

¼ teaspoon black pepper

Corn

8 cobs corn, husked

1 small handful of cilantro, chopped

1 teaspoon chili powder

Directions

Add all the ingredients for cashew sauce to a blender and blend until smooth.

Preheat the grill over medium-high heat.

Grill the corn cobs for 5 minutes per side until golden-brown.

Place the corn cobs on the serving plate and pour the cashew sauce on top.

Drizzle chili powder and cilantro on top.

Serve.

Nutritional Values

Calories: 201

Total Fat: 32.2 g

Saturated Fat: 2.4 g

Cholesterol: 110 mg

Sodium: 276 mg

Total Carbs: 25 g

Fiber: 0.9 g

Sugar: 1.4 g

Protein: 8.8 g

# Wild Rice Stuffed Portobelloss

Preparation Time: 10 minutes

Cooking Time: 1 hour 20 minutes

Servings: 6

Ingredients

1 cup wild rice

½ cup fresh basil

½ cup fresh mint

½ cup fresh parsley

1 tablespoon olive oil

1 tablespoon nutritional yeast

Juice of ½ lemon

Zest of 1 lemon

1 teaspoon honey

¾ cup pecans

Coconut oil, to grease

6 large portobello mushrooms

Salt and black pepper, to taste

Directions

Fill a saucepan with 3 cups of water and add wild rice to the water.

Add a pinch of sea salt to the water and cover the lid.

Cook the rice on a simmer for 50 minutes.

Drain the rice and remove the liquid.

Spread the pecans in a baking sheet and roast them for 8 minutes at 375°F in the oven.

Finely chop the pecans and keep them aside.

Now blend mint, basil, olive oil, parsley, lemon juice, nutritional yeast, honey, salt, and lemon zest in a blender.

Wash and clean the portobello mushroom caps and brush them with coconut oil.

Drizzle salt and black pepper over the mushrooms to season them.

Preheat the grill over medium-high heat.

Grill the mushroom caps for 6 minutes per side, under the lid.

Now stuff each mushroom cap with pesto, wild rice, and pecan.

Garnish with lemon zest.

Serve.

Nutritional Values

Calories: 219

Total Fat: 19.7 g

Saturated Fat: 18.6 g

Cholesterol: 141 mg

Sodium: 193 mg

Total Carbs: 23.7 g

Fiber: 0.2 g

Sugar: 1.3 g

Protein: 5.2 g

## Fung Tofu

Preparation Time: 10 minutes

Cooking Time: 12 minutes

Servings: 4

Ingredients

¼ cup soy sauce

½ cup black vinegar

1 tablespoon sesame oil

2 inches of fresh ginger peeled, minced

2 garlic cloves peeled, minced

¼ cup maple syrup

2 blocks firm tofu, pressed and cut into 4 slices

1 tablespoon sesame seeds

Directions

Mix soy sauce, sesame oil, black vinegar, ginger, garlic, maple syrup in a large bowl.

Toss in tofu and mix well to coat the slices well.

Keep the slices in a baking sheet and let them marinate for 1 hour.

Preheat the grill over medium-high heat.

Place the tofu slices on the grill and cook for 3 minutes per side.

Garnish with sesame seeds.

Serve.

Nutritional Values

Calories: 248

Total Fat: 15.7 g

Saturated Fat: 2.7 g

Cholesterol: 75 mg

Sodium: 94 mg

Total Carbs: 38.4 g

Fiber: 0.3 g

Sugar: 0.1 g

Protein: 14.1 g

## Thai Salad with Grilled Tofu

Preparation Time: 10 minutes

Cooking Time: 8 minutes

Servings: 4

Ingredients

Salad

¼ block tofu, cut into cubes

2 teaspoons soy sauce

1/8 red cabbage, sliced

½ carrot, peeled and sliced

3-inch piece cucumber, sliced

2 radishes, sliced

¼ red pepper, sliced

2 green onions, chopped

¼ cup cilantro, chopped

2 tablespoons peanuts, chopped

Dressing

½ garlic clove, minced

2 tablespoons rice vinegar

2 tablespoons peanut butter

½-inch piece ginger, minced

1 tablespoon soy sauce

1 tablespoon water

½ teaspoon sesame oil

½ teaspoon Sriracha

1 wedge lime

Directions

Add soy sauce and tofu to a bowl and mix well.

Leave the tofu for 15 minutes at room temperature.

Preheat the grill over medium heat.

Grill the tofu for 4 minutes per side.

Toss the remaining veggies and all other ingredients in a large bowl.

Mix well, then top the salad with grilled tofu.

Serve.

Nutritional Values

Calories: 301

Total Fat: 12.2 g

Saturated Fat: 2.4 g

Cholesterol: 110 mg

Sodium: 276 mg

Total Carbs: 12.5 g

Fiber: 0.9 g

Sugar: 1.4 g

Protein: 8.8 g

## Nori snack rolls

Preparation Time: 5 minutes
Cooking Time: 10 minutes

Servings: 4 rolls

Ingredients

2 tablespoons almond, cashew, peanut, or other nut butter

2 tablespoons tamari, or soy sauce

4 standard nori sheets

1 mushroom, sliced

1 tablespoon pickled ginger

½ cup grated carrots

Directions

Preheat the oven to 350°f.

Mix together the nut butter and tamari until smooth and very thick. Lay out a nori sheet, rough side up, the long way.

Spread a thin line of the tamari mixture on the far end of the nori sheet, from side to side. Lay the mushroom slices, ginger, and carrots in a line at the other end (the end closest to you).

Fold the vegetables inside the nori, rolling toward the tahini mixture, which will seal the roll. Repeat to make 4 rolls.

Put on a baking sheet and bake for 8 to 10 minutes, or until the rolls are slightly browned and crispy at the ends. Let the rolls cool for a few minutes, then slice each roll into 3 smaller pieces.

Nutrition: (1 roll) calories: 79; total fat: 5g; carbs: 6g; fiber: 2g; protein: 4g

Preparation Time: 15 minutes
Cooking Time: 20 minutes

Servings: 12 bites

Ingredients

½ cup panko bread crumbs

1 teaspoon paprika

1 teaspoon chipotle powder or ground cayenne pepper

1½ cups cold green pea risotto

Nonstick cooking spray

Directions

Preheat the oven to 425°f.

Line a baking sheet with parchment paper.

On a large plate, combine the panko, paprika, and chipotle powder. Set aside.

Roll 2 tablespoons of the risotto into a ball.

Gently roll in the bread crumbs, and place on the prepared baking sheet. Repeat to make a total of 12 balls.

Spritz the tops of the risotto bites with nonstick cooking spray and bake for 15 to 20 minutes, until they begin to brown. Cool completely before storing in a large airtight container in a single layer (add a piece of parchment paper for a second layer) or in a plastic freezer bag.

Nutrition: (6 bites): calories: 100; fat: 2g; protein: 6g; carbohydrates: 17g; fiber: 5g; sugar: 2g; sodium: 165mg

jicama and guacamole

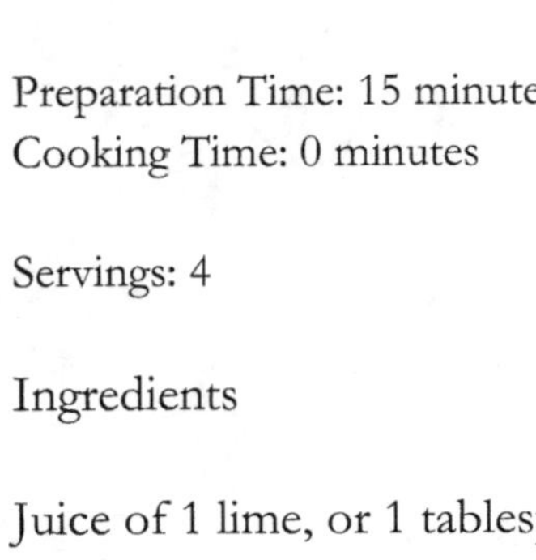

Preparation Time: 15 minutes
Cooking Time: 0 minutes

Servings: 4

Ingredients

Juice of 1 lime, or 1 tablespoon prepared lime juice

2 hass avocados, peeled, pits removed, and cut into cubes

½ teaspoon sea salt

½ red onion, minced

1 garlic clove, minced

¼ cup chopped cilantro (optional)

1 jicama bulb, peeled and cut into matchsticks

Directions


In a medium bowl, squeeze the lime juice over the top of the avocado and sprinkle with salt.

Lightly mash the avocado with a fork. Stir in the onion, garlic, and cilantro, if using.

Serve with slices of jicama to dip in guacamole.

To store, place plastic wrap over the bowl of guacamole and refrigerate. The guacamole will keep for about 2 days.

Preparation Time: 2 minutes
Cooking Time: 8 minutes

Servings: ½ cup

Ingredients

½ cup raw almonds, or sunflower seeds

2 tablespoons tamari, or soy sauce

1 teaspoon toasted sesame oil

Directions


Heat a dry skillet to medium-high heat, then add the almonds, stirring very frequently to keep them from burning. Once the almonds are toasted, 7 to 8 minutes for almonds, or 3 to 4 minutes for sunflower seeds, pour the tamari and sesame oil into the hot skillet and stir to coat.

You can turn off the heat, and as the almonds cool the tamari mixture will stick to and dry on the nuts.

Nutrition: (1 tablespoon) calories: 89; total fat: 8g; carbs: 3g; fiber: 2g; protein: 4g


## kale chips

Preparation Time: 5 minutes
Cooking Time: 25 minutes

Servings: 2

Ingredients

1 large bunch kale

1 tablespoon extra-virgin olive oil

½ teaspoon chipotle powder

½ teaspoon smoked paprika

¼ teaspoon salt

Directions

Preheat the oven to 275°f.

Line a large baking sheet with parchment paper. In a large bowl, stem the kale and tear it into bite-size pieces. Add the olive oil, chipotle powder, smoked paprika, and salt.

Toss the kale with tongs or your hands, coating each piece well.

Spread the kale over the parchment paper in a single layer.

Bake for 25 minutes, turning halfway through, until crisp.

Cool for 10 to 15 minutes before dividing and storing in 2 airtight containers.

Per serving: calories: 144; fat: 7g; protein: 5g; carbohydrates: 18g; fiber: 3g; sugar: 0g; sodium: 363mg

Peppers and hummus

Preparation Time: 15 minutes
Cooking Time: 0 minutes

Servings: 4

Ingredients

One 15-ounce can chickpeas, drained and rinsed

Juice of 1 lemon, or 1 tablespoon prepared lemon juice

¼ cup tahini

3 tablespoons olive oil

½ teaspoon ground cumin

1 tablespoon water

¼ teaspoon paprika

1 red bell pepper, sliced

1 green bell pepper, sliced

1 orange bell pepper, sliced

Directions


In a food processor, combine chickpeas, lemon juice, tahini, 2 tablespoons of the olive oil, the cumin, and water.

Process on high speed until blended, about 30 seconds. Scoop the hummus into a bowl and drizzle with the remaining tablespoon of olive oil. Sprinkle with paprika and serve with sliced bell peppers.

## Savory roasted chickpeas

Preparation Time: 5 minutes
Cooking Time: 25 minutes

Servings: 1 cup

Ingredients

1 (14-ounce) can chickpeas, rinsed and drained, or 1½ cups cooked

2 tablespoons tamari, or soy sauce

1 tablespoon nutritional yeast

1 teaspoon smoked paprika, or regular paprika

1 teaspoon onion powder

½ teaspoon garlic powder

Directions

Preheat the oven to 400°f.

Toss the chickpeas with all the other ingredients, and spread them out on a baking sheet. Bake for 20 to 25 minutes, tossing halfway through.

Bake these at a lower temperature, until fully dried and crispy, if you want to keep them longer.

You can easily double the batch, and if you dry them out they will keep about a week in an airtight container.

Nutrition: (¼ cup) calories: 121; total fat: 2g; carbs: 20g; fiber: 6g; protein: 8g


## Savory seed crackers

Preparation Time: 5 minutes
Cooking Time: 50 minutes

Servings: 20 crackers

Ingredients

¾ cup pumpkin seeds (pepitas)

½ cup sunflower seeds

½ cup sesame seeds

¼ cup chia seeds

1 teaspoon minced garlic (about 1 clove)

1 teaspoon tamari or soy sauce

1 teaspoon vegan worcestershire sauce

½ teaspoon ground cayenne pepper

½ teaspoon dried oregano

½ cup water

Directions


Preheat the oven to 325°f.

Line a rimmed baking sheet with parchment paper.

In a large bowl, combine the pumpkin seeds, sunflower seeds, sesame seeds, chia seeds, garlic, tamari, worcestershire sauce, cayenne, oregano, and water.

Transfer to the prepared baking sheet, spreading out to all sides.

Bake for 25 minutes. Remove the pan from the oven, and flip the seed "dough" over so the wet side is up. Bake for another 20 to 25 minutes, until the sides are browned.

Cool completely before breaking up into 20 pieces. Divide evenly among 4 glass jars and close tightly with lids.

Nutrition: (5 crackers): calories: 339; fat: 29g; protein: 14g; carbohydrates: 17g; fiber: 8g; sugar: 1g; sodium: 96mg


tomato and basil bruschetta

Preparation Time: 10 minutes
Cooking Time: 6 minutes

Servings: 12 bruschetta

Ingredients

3 tomatoes, chopped

¼ cup chopped fresh basil

1 tablespoon olive oil

Pinch of sea salt

1 baguette, cut into 12 slices

1 garlic clove, sliced in half

Directions

In a small bowl, combine the basil, salt, olive oil, and tomatoes and stir to mix. Set aside. Preheat the oven to 425°f.

Place the baguette slices in a single layer on a baking sheet and toast in the oven until brown, about 6 minutes.

Flip the bread slices over once during cooking. Remove from the oven and rub the bread on both sides with the sliced clove of -garlic.

Top with the tomato-basil mixture and serve immediately.

## Lemon coconut cilantro rolls

Preparation Time: 30 minutes • chill Preparation Time: 30 minutes

Servings: 16 pieces

Ingredients

½ cup fresh cilantro, chopped

1 cup sprouts (clover, alfalfa)

1 garlic clove, pressed

2 tablespoons ground brazil nuts or almonds

2 tablespoons flaked coconut

1 tablespoon coconut oil

Pinch cayenne pepper

Pinch sea salt

Pinch freshly ground black pepper

Zest and juice of 1 lemon

2 tablespoons ground flaxseed

1 to 2 tablespoons water

2 whole-grain wraps, or corn wraps

Directions

Put everything but the wraps in a food processor and pulse to combine. Or combine the ingredients in a large bowl. Add the water, if needed, to help the mix come together.

Spread the mixture out over each wrap, roll it up, and place it in the fridge for 30 minutes to set.

Remove the rolls from the fridge and slice each into 8 pieces to serve as appetizers or sides with a soup or stew.

Get the best flavor by buying whole raw brazil nuts or almonds, toasting them lightly in a dry skillet or toaster oven, and then grinding them in a coffee grinder.

Nutrition: (1 piece) calories: 66; total fat: 4g; carbs: 6g; fiber: 1g; protein: 2g

## Tamari Almonds

Preparation Time: 5 minutes
Cooking Time: 15 minutes

Servings: 8

Ingredients

1 pound raw almonds

3 tablespoons tamari or soy sauce

2 tablespoons extra-virgin olive oil

1 tablespoon nutritional yeast

1 to 2 teaspoons chili powder, to taste

Directions

Preheat the oven to 400°f.

Line a baking sheet with parchment paper.

In a medium bowl, combine the almonds, tamari, and olive oil until well coated.

Spread the almonds on the prepared baking sheet and roast for 10 to 15 minutes, until browned.

Cool for 10 minutes, then season with the nutritional yeast and chili powder.

Transfer to a glass jar and close tightly with a lid.

Per serving: calories: 364; fat: 32g; protein: 13g; carbohydrates: 13g; fiber: 7g; sugar: 3g; sodium: 381mg


stuffed cherry tomatoes

Preparation Time: 15 minutes
Cooking Time: 0 minutes

Servings: 6

Ingredients

2 pints cherry tomatoes, tops removed and centers scooped out

2 avocados, mashed

Juice of 1 lemon

½ red bell pepper, minced

4 green onions (white and green parts), finely minced

1 tablespoon minced fresh tarragon

Pinch of sea salt

Directions

Place the cherry tomatoes open-side up on a platter.

In a small bowl, -combine the avocado, lemon juice, bell pepper, scallions, tarragon, and salt.

Stir until well -combined. Scoop into the cherry tomatoes and serve immediately.

## Spicy black bean dip

Preparation Time: 10 minutes
Cooking Time: 0 minutes

Servings: 2 cups

Ingredients

1 (14-ounce) can black beans, drained and rinsed, or 1½ cups cooked

Zest and juice of 1 lime

1 tablespoon tamari, or soy sauce

¼ cup water

¼ cup fresh cilantro, chopped

1 teaspoon ground cumin

Pinch cayenne pepper

Directions


Put the beans in a food processor (best choice) or blender, along with the lime zest and juice, tamari, and about ¼ cup of water.

Blend until smooth, then blend in the cilantro, cumin, and cayenne.

If you don't have a blender or prefer a different consistency, simply transfer it to a bowl once the beans have been puréed and stir in the spices, instead of forcing the blender.

Nutrition: (1 cup) calories: 190; total fat: 1g; carbs: 35g; fiber: 12g; protein: 13g

# Baked Potato Chips

Preparation Time: 10 minutes
Cooking Time: 30 minutes

Servings: 4

Ingredients

1 large russet potato

1 teaspoon paprika

½ teaspoon garlic salt

¼ teaspoon vegan sugar

¼ teaspoon onion powder

¼ teaspoon chipotle powder or chili powder

⅛ teaspoon salt

⅛ teaspoon ground mustard

⅛ teaspoon ground cayenne pepper

1 teaspoon canola oil

⅛ teaspoon liquid smoke

Directions

Wash and peel the potato. Cut into thin, 1/10-inch slices (a mandoline slicer or the slicer blade in a food processor is helpful for consistently sized slices).

Fill a large bowl with enough very cold water to cover the potato. Transfer the potato slices to the bowl and soak for 20 minutes.

Preheat the oven to 400°f. Line a baking sheet with parchment paper.

In a small bowl, combine the paprika, garlic salt, sugar, onion powder, chipotle powder, salt, mustard, and cayenne.

Drain and rinse the potato slices and pat dry with a paper towel.

Transfer to a large bowl.

Add the canola oil, liquid smoke, and spice mixture to the bowl. Toss to coat.

Transfer the potatoes to the prepared baking sheet.

Bake for 15 minutes. Flip the chips over and bake for 15 minutes longer, until browned. Transfer the chips to 4 storage containers or large glass jars.

Let cool before closing the lids tightly.

Per serving: calories: 89; fat: 1g; protein: 2g; carbohydrates: 18g; fiber: 2g; sugar: 1g; sodium: 65mg


## Salsa Fresca

Preparation Time: 15 minutes
Cooking Time: 0 minutes

Servings: 4

Ingredients

3 large heirloom tomatoes or other fresh tomatoes, chopped

½ red onion, finely chopped

½ bunch cilantro, chopped

2 garlic cloves, minced

1 jalapeño, minced

Juice of 1 lime, or 1 tablespoon prepared lime juice

¼ cup olive oil

Sea salt

Whole-grain tortilla chips, for serving

Directions

In a small bowl, combine the tomatoes, onion, cilantro, garlic, jalapeño, lime juice, and olive oil and mix well. Allow to sit at room temperature for 15 minutes. Season with salt.

Serve with tortilla chips.

The salsa can be stored in an airtight container in the refrigerator for up to 1 week.

## Guacamole

Preparation Time: 10 minutes
Cooking Time: 0 minutes

Servings: 2

Ingredients

2 ripe avocados

2 garlic cloves, pressed

Zest and juice of 1 lime

1 teaspoon ground cumin

Pinch sea salt

Pinch freshly ground black pepper

Pinch cayenne pepper (optional)

Directions

Mash the avocados in a large bowl. Add the rest of the ingredients and stir to combine.

Try adding diced tomatoes (cherry are divine), chopped scallions or chives, chopped fresh cilantro or basil, lemon rather than lime, paprika, or whatever you think would taste good!

Nutrition: (1 cup) calories: 258; total fat: 22g; carbs: 18g; fiber: 11g; protein: 4g

## veggie hummus pinwheels

Preparation Time: 10 minutes
Cooking Time: 0 minutes

Servings: 3

Ingredients

3 whole-grain, spinach, flour, or gluten-free tortillas

3 large swiss chard leaves

¾ cup edamame hummus or prepared hummus

¾ cup shredded carrots

Directions

Lay 1 tortilla flat on a cutting board.

Place 1 swiss chard leaf over the tortilla. Spread ¼ cup of hummus over the swiss chard. Spread ¼ cup of carrots over the hummus. Starting at one end of the tortilla, roll tightly toward the opposite side.

Slice each roll up into 6 pieces. Place in a single-serving storage container.

Repeat with the remaining tortillas and filling and seal the lids.

Per serving: calories: 254; fat: 8g; protein: 10g; carbohydrates: 39g; fiber: 8g; sugar: 4g; sodium: 488mg

## Asian Lettuce Rolls

Preparation Time: 15 minutes
Cooking Time: 5 minutes

Servings: 4

Ingredients

2 ounces rice noodles

2 tablespoons chopped thai basil

2 tablespoons chopped cilantro

1 garlic clove, minced

1 tablespoon minced fresh ginger

Juice of ½ lime, or 2 teaspoons prepared lime juice

2 tablespoons soy sauce

1 cucumber, julienned

2 carrots, peeled and julienned

8 leaves butter lettuce

Directions


Cook the rice noodles according to package directions.

In a small bowl, whisk together the basil, cilantro, garlic, ginger, lime juice, and soy sauce. Toss with the cooked noodles, cucumber, and carrots.

Divide the mixture evenly among lettuce leaves and roll.

Secure with a toothpick and serve immediately.

## Sweet potato biscuits

Preparation Time: 60 minutes
Cooking Time: 10 minutes

Servings: 12 biscuits

Ingredients

1 medium sweet potato

3 tablespoons melted coconut oil, divided

1 tablespoon maple syrup

1 cup whole-grain flour

2 teaspoons baking powder

Pinch sea salt

Directions

Bake the sweet potato at 350°f for about 45 minutes, until tender.

Allow it to cool, then remove the flesh and mash.

Turn the oven up to 375°f and line a baking sheet with parchment paper or lightly grease it. Measure out 1 cup potato flesh.

In a medium bowl, combine the mashed sweet potato with 1½ tablespoons of the coconut oil and the maple syrup. Mix together the flour and baking powder in a separate medium bowl, then add the flour mixture to the potato mixture and blend well with a fork.

On a floured board, pat the mixture out into a ½-inch-thick circle and cut out 1-inch rounds, or simply drop spoonfuls of dough and pat them into rounds.

Put the rounds onto the prepared baking sheet. Brush the top of each with some of the remaining 1½ tablespoons melted coconut oil. Bake 10 minutes, or until lightly golden on top. Serve hot.

Nutrition: (1 biscuit) calories: 116; total fat: 4g; carbs: 19g; fiber: 3g; protein: 3g

Garlic toast

Preparation Time: 5 minutes
Cooking Time: 5 minutes

Servings: 1 slice

Ingredients

1 teaspoon coconut oil, or olive oil

Pinch sea salt

1 to 2 teaspoons nutritional yeast

1 small garlic clove, pressed, or ¼ teaspoon garlic powder

1 slice whole-grain bread

Directions

In a small bowl, mix together the oil, salt, nutritional yeast, and garlic.

You can either toast the bread and then spread it with the seasoned oil, or brush the oil on the bread and put it in a toaster oven to bake for 5 minutes.

If you're using fresh garlic, it's best to spread it onto the bread and then bake it.

Nutrition: (1 slice) calories: 138; total fat: 6g; carbs: 16g; fiber: 4g; protein: 7g

## Banana-nut bread bars

Preparation Time: 5 minutes
Cooking Time: 30 minutes

Servings: 9 bars

Ingredients

Nonstick cooking spray (optional)

2 large ripe bananas

1 tablespoon maple syrup

½ teaspoon vanilla extract

2 cups old-fashioned rolled oats

½ teaspoons salt

¼ cup chopped walnuts

Directions


Preheat the oven to 350°f. Lightly coat a 9-by-9-inch baking pan with nonstick cooking spray (if using) or line with parchment paper for oil-free baking.

In a medium bowl, mash the bananas with a fork. Add the maple syrup and vanilla extract and mix well. Add the oats, salt, and walnuts, mixing well.

Transfer the batter to the baking pan and bake for 25 to 30 minutes, until the top is crispy. Cool completely before slicing into 9 bars. Transfer to an airtight storage container or a large plastic bag.

Nutrition: (1 bar): calories: 73; fat: 1g; protein: 2g; carbohydrates: 15g; fiber: 2g; sugar: 5g; sodium: 129mg

## Apple crumble

Preparation Time: 20 minutes
Cooking Time: 25 minutes

Servings: 6

Ingredients

For the filling

4 to 5 apples, cored and chopped (about 6 cups)

½ cup unsweetened applesauce, or ¼ cup water

2 to 3 tablespoons unrefined sugar (coconut, date, sucanat, maple syrup)

1 teaspoon ground cinnamon

Pinch sea salt

For the crumble

2 tablespoons almond butter, or cashew or sunflower seed butter

2 tablespoons maple syrup

1½ cups rolled oats

½ cup walnuts, finely chopped

½ teaspoon ground cinnamon

2 to 3 tablespoons unrefined granular sugar (coconut, date, sucanat)

Directions

Preheat the oven to 350°f. Put the apples and applesauce in an 8-inch-square baking dish, and sprinkle with the sugar, cinnamon, and salt. Toss to combine.

In a medium bowl, mix together the nut butter and maple syrup until smooth and creamy. Add the oats, walnuts, cinnamon, and sugar and stir to coat, using your hands if necessary. (if you have a small food processor, pulse the oats and walnuts together before adding them to the mix.)

Sprinkle the topping over the apples, and put the dish in the oven.

Bake for 20 to 25 minutes, or until the fruit is soft and the topping is lightly browned.

Nutrition: calories: 356; total fat: 17g; carbs: 49g; fiber: 7g; protein: 7g

## Cashew-Chocolate Truffles

Preparation Time: 15 minutes
Cooking Time: 0 minutes • plus 1 hour to set

Servings: 12 truffles

Ingredients

1 cup raw cashews, soaked in water overnight

¾ cup pitted dates

2 tablespoons coconut oil

1 cup unsweetened shredded coconut, divided

1 to 2 tablespoons cocoa powder, to taste

Directions

In a food processor, combine the cashews, dates, coconut oil, ½ cup of shredded coconut, and cocoa powder. Pulse until fully incorporated; it will resemble chunky cookie dough. Spread the remaining ½ cup of shredded coconut on a plate.

Form the mixture into tablespoon-size balls and roll on the plate to cover with the shredded coconut. Transfer to a parchment paper–lined plate or baking sheet. Repeat to make 12 truffles.

Place the truffles in the refrigerator for 1 hour to set. Transfer the truffles to a storage container or freezer-safe bag and seal.

Nutrition: (1 truffle): calories 238: fat: 18g; protein: 3g; carbohydrates: 16g; fiber: 4g; sugar: 9g; sodium: 9mg

Preparation Time: 20 minutes
Cooking Time: 20 minutes

Servings: 12 cupcakes

Ingredients

3 medium bananas

1 cup non-dairy milk

2 tablespoons almond butter

1 teaspoon apple cider vinegar

1 teaspoon pure vanilla extract

1¼ cups whole-grain flour

½ cup rolled oats

¼ cup coconut sugar (optional)

1 teaspoon baking powder

½ teaspoon baking soda

½ cup unsweetened cocoa powder

¼ cup chia seeds, or sesame seeds

Pinch sea salt

¼ cup dark chocolate chips, dried cranberries, or raisins (optional)

Directions

Preheat the oven to 350°f. Lightly grease the cups of two 6-cup muffin tins or line with paper muffin cups.

Put the bananas, milk, almond butter, vinegar, and vanilla in a blender and purée until smooth. Or stir together in a large bowl until smooth and creamy.

Put the flour, oats, sugar (if using), baking powder, baking soda, cocoa powder, chia seeds, salt, and chocolate chips in another large bowl, and stir to combine. Mix together the wet and dry ingredients, stirring as little as possible. Spoon into muffin cups, and bake for 20 to 25 minutes. Take the cupcakes out of the oven and let them cool fully before taking out of the muffin tins, since they'll be very moist.

Nutrition: (1 cupcake) calories: 215; total fat: 6g; carbs: 39g; fiber: 9g; protein: 6g

## Minty fruit salad

Preparation Time: 15 minutes
Cooking Time: 5 minutes

Servings: 4

Ingredients

¼ cup lemon juice (about 2 small lemons)

4 teaspoons maple syrup or agave syrup

2 cups chopped pineapple

2 cups chopped strawberries

2 cups raspberries

1 cup blueberries

8 fresh mint leaves

Directions

Beginning with 1 mason jar, add the ingredients in this order:

1 tablespoon of lemon juice, 1 teaspoon of maple syrup, ½ cup of pineapple, ½ cup of strawberries, ½ cup of raspberries, ¼ cup of blueberries, and 2 mint leaves.

Repeat to fill 3 more jars. Close the jars tightly with lids.

Place the airtight jars in the refrigerator for up to 3 days.

Per serving: calories: 138; fat: 1g; protein: 2g; carbohydrates: 34g; fiber: 8g; sugar: 22g; sodium: 6mg


## Mango coconut cream pie

Preparation Time: 20 minutes • chill Preparation Time: 30 minutes

Servings: 8

Ingredients

For the crust

½ cup rolled oats

1 cup cashews

1 cup soft pitted dates

For the filling

1 cup canned coconut milk

½ cup water

2 large mangos, peeled and chopped, or about 2 cups frozen chunks

½ cup unsweetened shredded coconut

Directions


Put all the crust ingredients in a food processor and pulse until it holds together. If you don't have a food processor, chop everything as finely as possible and use ½ cup cashew or almond butter in place of half the cashews. Press the mixture down firmly into an 8-inch pie or springform pan.

Put the all filling ingredients in a blender and purée until smooth (about 1 minute). It should be very thick, so you may have to stop and stir until it's smooth.

Pour the filling into the crust, use a rubber spatula to smooth the top, and put the pie in the freezer until set, about 30 minutes. Once frozen, it should be set out for about 15 minutes to soften before serving.

Top with a batch of coconut whipped cream scooped on top of the pie once it's set. Finish it off with a sprinkling of toasted shredded coconut.

Nutrition: (1 slice) calories: 427; total fat: 28g; carbs: 45g; fiber: 6g; protein: 8g

## Kale Chips

Servings: 4

Preparation Time: 25 Minutes

Calories: 25.1

Protein: 1.7 Grams

Fat: 0.4 Grams

Carbs: 5 Grams

Ingredients:

1 Bunch Kale

1 Spritz Olive Oil

Directions:

Heat your oven to 250, and then wash your kale before patting it dry.

Arrange your kale on a prepared baking sheet, making sure your kale doesn't overlap. Spray it down with olive oil, and then season with salt.

Cook for twenty minutes.

Zucchini Brownies

Servings: 24

Preparation Time: 45 Minutes

Calories: 138

Protein: 1.5 Grams

Fat: 4.8 Grams

Carbs: 21.9 Grams

Ingredients;

2 Cups Flour

1 ½ Cups Vegan Sugar

1 Teaspoon Baking Soda

1 Teaspoon Sea Salt, Fine

½ Cup Cocoa, Unsweetened

2 Tablespoons Vanilla Extract, Pure

½ Cup Oil

2 Cups Zucchini, Peeled & Grated

Directions:

Mix your cocoa, salt, flour, sugar and baking soda together.

Add in your oil, vanilla and zucchini, mixing well.

Bake at 350 in a nine by thirteen inch pan until done.

# Mint Chocolate Chip Sorbet

Preparation Time: 5 minutes
Cooking Time: 0 minutes

Servings: 1

Ingredients

1 frozen banana

1 tablespoon almond butter, or peanut butter, or other nut or seed butter

2 tablespoons fresh mint, minced

¼ cup or less non-dairy milk (only if needed)

2 to 3 tablespoons non-dairy chocolate chips, or cocoa nibs

2 to 3 tablespoons goji berries (optional)

Directions


Put the banana, almond butter, and mint in a food processor or blender and purée until smooth.

Add the non-dairy milk if needed to keep blending (but only if needed, as this will make the texture less solid). Pulse the chocolate chips and goji berries (if using) into the mix so they're roughly chopped up.

Nutrition: calories: 212; total fat: 10g; carbs: 31g; fiber: 4g; protein: 3g

# Peach-mango crumble  (pressure cooker)

Preparation Time: 10 minutes • pressure: 6 minutes • total: 21 minutes • pressure level: high • release: quick

Serves 4-6

Ingredients

3 cups chopped fresh or frozen peaches

3 cups chopped fresh or frozen mangos

4 tablespoons unrefined sugar or pure maple syrup, divided

1 cup gluten-free rolled oats

½ cup shredded coconut, sweetened or unsweetened

2 tablespoons coconut oil or vegan margarine

Directions

Preparing the ingredients. In a 6- to 7-inch round baking dish, toss together the peaches, mangos, and 2 tablespoons of sugar. In a food processor, combine the oats, coconut, coconut oil, and remaining 2 tablespoons of sugar. Pulse until combined. (if you use maple syrup, you'll need less coconut oil. Start with just the syrup and add oil if the mixture isn't sticking together.) Sprinkle the oat mixture over the fruit mixture.

Cover the dish with aluminum foil. Put a trivet in the bottom of your electric pressure cooker's cooking pot and pour in a cup or two of water. Using a foil sling or silicone helper handles, lower the pan onto the trivet.

High pressure for 6 minutes. Close and lock the lid, and select high pressure for 6 minutes.

Pressure release. Once the cook time is complete, quick release the pressure. Unlock and remove the lid.

Let cool for a few minutes before carefully lifting out the dish with oven mitts or tongs. Scoop out portions to serve.

Nutrition: calories: 321; total fat: 18g; protein: 4g; sodium: 2mg; fiber: 7g

## Zesty orange-cranberry energy bites

Preparation Time: 10 minutes • chill Preparation Time: 15 minutes

Servings: 12 bites

Ingredients

2 tablespoons almond butter, or cashew or sunflower seed butter

2 tablespoons maple syrup, or brown rice syrup

¾ cup cooked quinoa

¼ cup sesame seeds, toasted

1 tablespoon chia seeds

½ teaspoon almond extract, or vanilla extract

Zest of 1 orange

1 tablespoon dried cranberries

¼ cup ground almonds

Directions

In a medium bowl, mix together the nut or seed butter and syrup until smooth and creamy. Stir in the rest of the ingredients, and mix to make sure the consistency is holding together in a ball. Form the mix into 12 balls.

Place them on a baking sheet lined with parchment or waxed paper and put in the fridge to set for about 15 minutes.

If your balls aren't holding together, it's likely because of the moisture content of your cooked quinoa. Add more nut or seed butter mixed with syrup until it all sticks together.

Nutrition: (1 bite) calories: 109; total fat: 7g; carbs: 11g; fiber: 3g; protein: 3g

## Irish Bombay Potatoes

Preparation Time: 5 minutes
Cooking Time: 30 minutes
Servings: 4

5 Ingredients

35 oz potato, peeled

2 tbsp curry paste

2 tbsp tomato paste

½ cup basil, fresh

1 garlic clove

What you'll need from the store cupboard

1tbsp salt

4 tbsp oil

2 tbsp curry powder

2 tbsp white vinegar

Directions

Heat your oven to 3900F.

Quarter the peeled potatoes and place them in a mixing bowl.

Add curry paste, tomato paste, salt, oil, curry powder then mix until the potatoes ate well coated.

Layer the potatoes on your oven tray and bake them for fifteen minutes.

Add fresh basil and garlic five minutes before the end of cooking. Mix well making sure the spices are well mixed in.

Serve with dips or as a side dish. Enjoy.

Nutrition Facts Nutrition:

Calories 288, Total Fat 14g, Saturated Fat 1g, Total Carbs 33g, Net Carbs 25g, Protein 7g, Sugar 1g, Fiber 7g, Sodium 670mg, Potassium 1129mg

## Healthy Mashed Sweet Potato

Preparation Time: 5 minutes
Cooking Time: 20 minutes
Servings: 2

5 Ingredients

2 sweet potatoes, peeled and chopped

2 garlic cloves

1 thumb ginger, fresh

1 chili pepper

1 handful coriander, fresh

What you'll need from the store cupboard

6 tbsp olive oil

½ juiced lime

Directions

Add sweet potatoes to boiling and salted water in a saucepan. Let the sweet potatoes cook for twenty minutes.

Meanwhile, add olive oil to a small pan. Add chopped garlic cloves and ginger.

Make an incision on the chili pepper or make four incisions on the chili pepper if you like your food spicier.

Let the three fry in oil for some few minutes.

When the sweet potatoes are cooked, poke them with a knife to make sure they are fully soft.

Add the potatoes in the pan and use a spoon to remove the garlic, ginger and chili pieces from the oil. The heat should be off.

Mash all them together until smooth.

Serve with coriander and lime juice. Enjoy.

Nutrition Facts Nutrition:

Calories 503, Total Fat 42g, Saturated Fat 5g, Total Carbs 31g, Net Carbs 27g, Protein 2g, Sugar 6g, Fiber 4g, Sodium 76mg, Potassium 532mg

## Spinach Tomato Quesadilla

Preparation Time: 5 minutes
Cooking Time: 10 minutes
Servings: 2

5 Ingredients

2 whole-grain tortillas

½ cup cheddar cheese, sliced

1 cup mozzarella cheese, sliced

1 tomato

1 ½ cup spinach

What you'll need from the store cupboard

1 tbsp homemade pesto

Directions

Spread a layer of homemade pesto over half tortilla.

Add a cheese layer on the tortilla.

Slice the tomato and a layer on the cheese.

Add a layer of spinach on top then finally another cheese layer

Fold the other half of the tortilla on top.

Place the tortilla on a hot pan, cover the pan and heat for four minutes on each side. The cheese should have melted.

Serve and enjoy.

Nutrition Facts Nutrition:

Calories 386, Total Fat 19g, Saturated Fat 9g, Total Carbs 26g, Net Carbs 20g, Protein 23g, Sugar 3g, Fiber 5g, Sodium 863mg, Potassium 254mg

## Lentil Tacos

Preparation Time: 5 minutes
Cooking Time: 15 minutes
Servings: 6

5 Ingredients

1 onion, diced

2 garlic cloves, diced

1 cup brown lentils, cooked

2 tbsp burrito seasoning

2 taco shells

What you'll need from the store cupboard

2 tbsp olive oil

4 cups of water

6 tbsp salsa

1 ½ cups mixed salad

½ cup cherry tomatoes, sliced

Directions

Heat olive oil in a saucepan and fry the onions until soft.

Add diced garlic then drain the lentils and add them.

Add seasoning and water then stir well. Cook until all water has evaporated.

Meanwhile, put the taco shells in the oven to cook for three minutes.

Layer the lentils at the bottom followed by cheese if you desire, salsa, mixed salad and finally the cherry tomatoes.

Serve and enjoy.

Nutrition Facts Nutrition:

Calories 239, Total Fat 13g, Saturated Fat 5g, Total Carbs 20g, Net Carbs 14g, Protein 9g, Sugar 2g, Fiber 5g, Sodium 350mg, Potassium 296mg

## Flawless Feta and Spinach Pancakes

Preparation Time: 10 minutes
Cooking Time: 20 minutes
Servings: 4

5 Ingredients

17 oz spinach, frozen

1 cup flour

2 eggs

1cup milk

5 oz feta cheese

What you'll need from the store cupboard

2 tbsp butter

Salt to taste

Directions

Heat a pot on medium heat then add the frozen spinach. Stir frequently to deforest the spinach quickly.

Add flour, eggs, and milk in a mixing bowl then use a hand mixer to mix until there are no lumps.

Add more milk until you achieve the desired consistency.

Heat a nonstick skillet over medium heat.

Melt butter and pour the mixture on the pan — Fry for four minutes on each side.

Layer the pancake on a plate then pour the heated spinach on one half of the pancake.

Layer cheese slices on the spinach then fold the pancake.

Serve and enjoy.

Nutrition Facts Nutrition:

Calories 361, Total Fat 18g, Saturated Fat 10g, Total Carbs 33g, Net Carbs 27g, Protein 17g, Sugar 5g, Fiber 4g, Sodium 593mg, Potassium 583mg

## Eggplant Curry

Preparation Time: 5 minutes
Cooking Time: 30 minutes
Servings: 2

5 Ingredients

1 aubergine

1 red onion

2 garlic cloves, crushed

1 cup tomatoes, chopped

1 ½ cups of coconut milk

What you'll need from the store cupboard

2 tbsp olive oil

1 tbsp curry powder

1 tbsp turmeric

1 tbsp coriander

Salt and pepper to taste

1 tbsp sugar

Directions

Cook the rice according to the package directions

Fry the aubergine in olive oil over high heat for four minutes. Stir well so that it doesn't burn.

Add onions then lower the heat to medium. Cook for five minutes.

Stir in garlic, curry powder, turmeric, and coriander — Cook for four minutes.

Add tomatoes and milk then season with salt and pepper to taste.

Simmer until your desired consistency is achieved.

Add sugar for a little sweetener if you desire.

Serve and enjoy

Nutrition Facts Nutrition:

Calories 379, Total Fat 27g, Saturated Fat 14g, Total Carbs 27g, Net Carbs 17g, Protein 3g, Sugar 10g, Fiber 9g, Sodium 749mg, Potassium 663mg

## Dumplings

Preparation Time: 5 minutes
Cooking Time: 15 minutes
Servings: 6

Ingredients

1 cup all-purpose flour

1 tbsp white sugar

1 tbsp margarine

½ cup milk

What you'll need from store cupboard

2 tbsp baking powder

½ tbsp salt

Directions

Stir together flour, sugar, baking powder, and salt in a bowl (medium-size).

Cut in margarine until crumbly.

Add milk and stir to make dough soft.

Drop the dough into a boiling stew by spoonfuls then cover and simmer for about 15 minutes. Do not lift lid.

Serve.

Nutritional Facts Per Servings

Calories: 105 total fat: 2.4g saturated fat: 1g total carbs: 18g net carbs: 17.4g protein: 2.8g sugars: 2g dietary fiber: 0.6g sodium: 386mg potassium: 54mg

## Potato Dumplings II

Preparation Time: 10 minutes
Cooking Time: 20 minutes
Servings: 6

Ingredients

1 cup instant mashed potato flakes

1 cup hot water

¾ cup all-purpose flour

What you'll need from store cupboard

1 tbsp salt

2 eggs

Directions

Put potato flakes, salt, and water in a mixing bowl. Mix and allow to cool for about 10 minutes.

Add eggs and flour and stir.

Knead the dough on a surface (lightly floured) until not sticky. Make 6 dumplings from the dough.

Boil water in a large saucepan then drop in the dumplings.

Boil for about 20 minutes until dumplings rise to the top.

Remove and drain the dumplings.

Nutritional Facts Per Servings

Calories: 108 total fat: 1.9g saturated fat: 1g total carbs: 18.1g net carbs: 17.1g protein: 4.3g sugars: 0g Dietary fiber: 1g sodium: 419mg potassium: 142mg

## Grandma's Noodles II

Prep time 2 hours: Cook Preparation Time: 30 minutes
Servings: 4

Ingredients

2 tbsp milk

1 cup all-purpose (sifted)

What you'll need from store cupboard

1 beaten egg

½ tbsp salt

Optional: ½ tbsp baking powder

Directions

Combine egg, milk, and salt then add flour and mix. ( add baking powder for thicker noodles before mixing).

Separate the mixture into two balls.

Roll out dough then let sit for about 20 minutes.

Cut the dough into strips then spread to dry. Dust with flour and let dry for about 2 hours.

Drop the strips into hot soup and cook for about 10 minutes.

Serve and enjoy.

Nutritional Facts Nutrition:

Calories: 136 total fat: 1.7g saturated fat: 1g total carbs: 24.5g net carbs: 23.7g protein: 5.1g sugars: 1g dietary fiber: 0.8g sodium: 373mg potassium: 62mg

# Pasta with Fresh Tomato Sauce

Preparation Time: 15 minutes
Cooking Time: 10 minutes
Servings: 8

Ingredients

16 oz dry penne pasta

8 Roma plum tomatoes, diced

¼ cup fresh basil, finely chopped

½ cup Italian dressing

What you'll need from store cupboard

¼ cup parmesan cheese (grated)

¼ cup red onion (diced)

Salt to taste

Directions

Boil lightly salted water in a large pot then add penne pasta and cook for about 10 minutes until al dente. Now drain.

Transfer the cooked pasta into a large bowl and toss with tomatoes, basil, Italian dressing, parmesan cheese, and red onion.

Serve and enjoy.

Nutrition Facts Nutrition:

Calories: 257 total fat: 3.1g saturated fat: 1g total carbs: 46.9g net carbs: 43.5g protein: 9.8g sugars: 3g dietary fiber: 3.4g sodium: 248mg potassium: 236mg

# Penne with Spring Vegetables

Preparation Time: 10 minutes
Cooking Time: 15 minutes
Servings: 4

Ingredients

1 lb trimmed fresh asparagus (½ inch pieces)

8 oz trimmed sugar snap peas

8 oz dry penne pasta

What you'll need from store cupboard

½ cup parmesan cheese (grated)

3 tbsp olive oil

Pepper and salt to taste

Directions

Boil lightly salted water in a large pot then add asparagus and cook for about 2 minutes.

Add peas and cook for an additional 2 minutes. Transfer to a set-aside bowl (large).

Add pasta to the boiling water then cook for about 8-10 minutes until al dente. Now drain.

Add pasta to the bowl with asparagus then toss with parmesan, olive oil, pepper, and salt.

Serve.

Nutritional Facts Nutrition:

Calories: 383 total fat: 14.4g saturated fat: 3g total carbs: 50.4g net carbs: 44.8g Protein: 15.2g sugars: 4g dietary fiber: 5.6g sodium: 158mg potassium: 347mg

## One Pan Mexican Rice

Preparation Time: 10 minutes
Cooking Time: 30 minutes
Servings: 6

5 Ingredients

1 cup brown rice, quick cook

1 can kidney beans drain and rinse

1 can corn, drained

1 can tomato sauce

1 tbsp adobo seasoning

What you'll need from the store cupboard

1 ½ cup water

½ tbsp oregano, dried

½ tbsp salt

⅛ tbsp black pepper

1 tbsp cumin

1 tbsp garlic powder

1 tbsp onion powder

Directions

Add all the ingredients to a nonstick skillet.

Bring to boil.

Reduce heat to medium and cover the skillet. Simmer until the rice is soft and all the liquid is absorbed.

Remove the lid and reduce heat to low. Stir occasionally until the rice is completely cooked.

Serve and enjoy.

Nutrition Facts Nutrition:

Calories 153, Total Fat 1g, Saturated Fat 0g, Total Carbs 33g, Net Carbs 28g, Protein 5g, Sugar 7g, Fiber 3g, Sodium 794mg, Potassium 542 mg

## Red Rice and Beans

Preparation Time: 10 minutes
Cooking Time: 60 minutes
Servings: 6

5 Ingredients

¼ tbsp red pepper flakes

1 can tomatoes, diced

2 cups brown rice, long grain

1 can black beans, rinsed

¼ cup cilantro

What you'll need from the store cupboard

¼ cup extra virgin oil

1 onion, diced

1 bell pepper, diced

2 garlic cloves

1 tbsp cumin, ground

4 cups vegetable broth

Directions

Add oil in your heavy-bottomed skillet then sauté onions for three minutes.

Add bell pepper and sauté for four minutes.

Add garlic, ground cumin, and pepper flakes. Sauté for a minute.

Add tomatoes and stir cook for five minutes.

Add brown rice and vegetable broth then stir to mix everything. Bring to boil then reduce heat to low. Simmer until the brown rice is cooked through.

Stir in cilantro and beans then let rest for five minutes.

Serve and enjoy

Nutrition Facts Nutrition:

Calories 445, Total Fat 11g, Saturated Fat 1g, Total Carbs 74g, Net Carbs 62g, Protein 12g, Sugar 1g, Fiber 5g, Sodium 645mg, Potassium 617mg

## Mexican Brown Rice

Preparation Time: 10 minutes
Cooking Time: 10 minutes
Servings: 5

5 Ingredients

1 ½ cups corn, fresh

1 can black beans, drain and rinse

3 cups brown rice, whole grain and ready to serve

1 cup jarred salsa

Cilantro for garnish

What you'll need from the store cupboard

1 tbsp chili powder

Directions

Preheat your nonstick skillet over medium heat.

Add corn and beans then cook until tender.

Add rice and chili powder then stir to combine. Stir cook for three minutes.

Stir in jarred salsa and cook until everything is warmed through.

Remove from heat and let rest for ten minutes. Garnish with cilantro.

Serve and enjoy.

Nutrition Facts Nutrition:

Calories 215, Total Fat 3g, Saturated Fat 1g, Total Carbs 42g, Net Carbs 35g, Protein 8g, Sugar 2g, Fiber 7g, Sodium 458mg, Potassium 417mg

## Black Beans and Rice

Preparation Time: 5 minutes
Cooking Time: 30 minutes
Servings: 10

5 Ingredients

1 onion, chopped

2 garlic cloves, minced

¾ cup white rice

1 /4 tbsp cayenne pepper

3 ½ cups black beans, canned, drained and rinsed

What you'll need from the store cupboard

1 tbsp olive oil

1 ½ cup vegetable broth, low sodium, and low fat

1 tbsp cumin, ground

Directions

Add olive oil in a stockpot over medium heat. Add onions and garlic. Saute for four minutes.

Add rice and saute for two more minutes.

Add vegetable broth and bring to boil. Cover, lower heat to medium and cook for twenty more minutes.

Add cumin, cayenne pepper, and black beans then stir.

Serve and enjoy

Nutrition Facts Nutrition:

Calories 140, Total Fat 1g, Saturated Fat 0g, Total Carbs 27g, Net Carbs 19g, Protein 6g, Sugar 1g, Fiber 6g, Sodium 354mg, Potassium 298mg

## Coconut Rice with Black Beans

Preparation Time: 5 minutes
Cooking Time: 25 minutes
Servings: 6

5 Ingredients

½ shallot, minced

1 cup jasmine rice, uncooked

¾ cup coconut milk

1 pinch nutmeg, ground

1 can black beans, drained and rinsed

What you'll need from the store cupboard

1 tbsp butter

1 cup water

Directions

Melt butter in a saucepan over medium-high heat. Sauté until the shallots are translucent.

Add jasmine rice and stir until the rice is evenly coated with melted butter.

Add coconut milk and water. Season with nutmeg then bring to boil over high heat.

Reduce to medium and simmer until rice is tender, and there is no liquid.

Stir in the beans and cook until hot.

Serve and enjoy.

Nutrition Facts Nutrition:

Calories 190, Total Fat 8g, Saturated Fat 7g, Total Carbs 27g, Net Carbs 25g, Protein 3g, Sugar 0g, Fiber 1g, Sodium 19mg, Potassium 78mg

## Quick Black Beans and Rice

Preparation Time: 5 minutes
Cooking Time: 15 minutes
Servings: 6

5 Ingredients

1 onion, chopped

1 can black beans, undrained

1 can stewed tomatoes

1 tbsp oregano, dried

1 ½ brown rice, uncooked

What you'll need from the store cupboard

1 tbsp vegetable oil

½ tbsp garlic powder

Directions

Heat vegetable oil in a large saucepan over medium heat.

Add onion and sauté until tender.

Add beans, stewed tomatoes, dried oregano, and garlic. Bring to boil.

Stir in brown rice, reduce heat to low. Simmer for five minutes and remove from heat.

Let rest for five minutes then serve. Enjoy.

Nutrition Facts Nutrition:

Calories 271, Total Fat 5g, Saturated Fat 0g, Total Carbs 48g, Net Carbs 35g, Protein 10g, Sugar 5g, Fiber 9g, Sodium 552mg, Potassium 260mg

## Rosemary Cider Mocktail

Preparation Time: 10 minutes

Cooking Time: 0 minutes

Servings: 1

Ingredients

4 oz apple cider

4 oz club soda

1 tablespoon rosemary syrup

1 sprig fresh rosemary

Directions

Add club soda, cider, and simple syrup in a jug.

Pour into the serving glasses and garnish with rosemary sprig.

Serve.

Nutritional Values

Calories: 64

Total Fat: 0 g

Saturated Fat: 0 g

Cholesterol: 0 mg

Sodium: 54 mg

Total Carbs: 14.1 g

Sugar: 0.3 g

Fiber: 0.4 g

Protein: 0.4 g

# Strawberry Lemon Mocktail

Preparation Time: 10 minutes

Cooking Time: 0 minutes

Servings: 1

Ingredients

2 strawberries

2 leaves fresh basil

1 teaspoon lemon zest

¾ oz strawberry shrub

3 ice cubes

5 oz cold plain seltzer

Directions

Dump all the ingredients into the cocktail shaker.

Shake the mocktail mixture for 1 minute.

Serve.

Nutritional Values

Calories: 61

Total Fat: 1.3 g

Saturated Fat: 0.7 g

Cholesterol: 3 mg

Sodium: 23 mg

Total Carbs: 18.5 g

Sugar: 11.1 g

Fiber: 0.3 g

Protein: 0.3 g

## White Russian Drink

Preparation Time: 10 minutes

Cooking Time: 0 minutes

Servings: 2

Ingredients

Cashew Cream

1 cup raw cashews

2 cups water

2 tablespoons maple syrup

2 teaspoons vanilla extract

Cocktail

1 oz vodka

1 oz Kahlua

2 oz cashew cream, to serve

# Directions

Throw all the ingredients for the cashew cream into a blender and blend well.

Dump all the ingredients into the cocktail shaker.

Shake the mocktail mixture for 1 minute.

Garnish with cashew cream.

Serve.

Nutritional Values

Calories: 19

Total Fat: 0.4 g

Saturated Fat: 0 g

Cholesterol: 0 mg

Sodium: 52 mg

Total Carbs: 24.8 g

Sugar: 2.4 g

Fiber: 1.4 g

Protein: 0.4 g

# Red Hot Chocolate

Preparation Time: 10 minutes

Cooking Time: 0 minutes

Servings: 2

Ingredients

2 cups almond milk

½ beet, cooked and grated

3 tablespoons raw cacao powder

3–6 dates, pitted and chopped

½ teaspoon vanilla extract

¼ teaspoon ground cinnamon

1 pinch sea salt

Coconut cream, to serve

Shaved dark chocolate, to serve

Directions

Dump all the hot chocolate ingredients into a blender jug.

Blend the chocolate mixture for 2 minutes.

Transfer this hot chocolate mixture to a saucepan and heat it for 5 minutes.

Divide the red velvet hot chocolate into the serving mugs.

Garnish with dark chocolate and coconut cream.

Serve.

Nutritional Values

Calories: 98

Total Fat: 1.5 g

Saturated Fat: 0 g

Cholesterol: 0 mg

Sodium: 94 mg

Total Carbs: 31.5 g

Sugar: 1.3 g

Fiber: 0.1 g

Protein: 10 g

## Blackberry Mint Beverage

Preparation Time: 10 minutes

Cooking Time: 0 minutes

Servings: 2

Ingredients

1 ½ cups fresh blackberries

½ tablespoon coconut sugar

½ teaspoon ground cinnamon

¼ teaspoon ground nutmeg

2 cups apple cider

3 sprigs fresh thyme

Directions

Dump all the mint beverage ingredients into a large saucepan.

Cook the mixture for 5 minutes on a simmer.

Strain the cooked lemon beverage through a fine sieve.

Serve.

Nutritional Values

Calories: 121

Total Fat: 1.2 g

Saturated Fat: 0.7 g

Cholesterol: 3 mg

Sodium: 84 mg

Total Carbs: 7.5 g

Sugar: 6 g

Fiber: 0.3 g

Protein: 0.6 g

## Almond Hot Cocoa Drink

Preparation Time: 10 minutes

Cooking Time: 5 minutes

Servings: 2

Ingredients

2 cups almond milk

3 tablespoons natural cocoa powder

2 tablespoons almond butter

20 raw almonds, finely chopped

Directions

Dump all the ingredients into a saucepan.

Stir the mixture for 5 minutes on low heat.

Serve.

Nutritional Values

Calories: 115

Total Fat: 1.1 g

Saturated Fat: 0.4 g

Cholesterol: 2 mg

Sodium: 24 mg

Total Carbs: 24.1 g

Sugar: 1.3 g

Fiber: 0.3 g

Protein: 2.5 g

Preparation Time: 10 minutes

Cooking Time: 5 minutes

Servings: 2

Ingredients

2 cups almond milk

2 tablespoons cacao or cocoa powder

3 tablespoons vegan mini chocolate chips

1 teaspoon vanilla extract

1 teaspoon cinnamon powder

½ teaspoon ginger powder

¼ teaspoon nutmeg powder

Toppings

Cinnamon

Vegan whipped cream

Vegan marshmallows

Directions

Dump all the ginger chocolate ingredients into a large saucepan.

Cook the mixture for 5 minutes on a simmer.

Garnish with desired toppings.

Serve.

Nutritional Values

Calories: 185

Total Fat: 0.1 g

Saturated Fat: 0 g

Cholesterol: 0 mg

Sodium: 144 mg

Total Carbs: 6.1 g

Sugar: 3.5 g

Fiber: 0.1 g

Protein: 0.1 g

Preparation Time: 10 minutes

Cooking Time: 5 minutes

Servings: 2

Ingredients

1 (25.4 oz) bottle red wine

2 tablespoons brown rum

2 oranges, sliced

Juice of 2 oranges

5 cloves

2 cinnamon sticks

2-star aniseed

½ cup brown sugar

Directions

Dump all the wine ingredients into a large saucepan.

Cook the mixture for 5 minutes on a simmer.

Strain the cooked mulled wine through a fine sieve.

Serve.

Nutritional Values

Calories: 109

Total Fat: 12 g

Saturated Fat: 03 g

Cholesterol: 01 mg

Sodium: 10 mg

Total Carbs: 23.6 g

Sugar: 2 g

Fiber: 0 g

Protein: 10 g

## Hibiscus Latte

Preparation Time: 10 minutes

Cooking Time: 5 minutes

Servings: 1

**Ingredients**

½ cup water

2 drops rose water

2-inch cube ginger

2 hibiscus tea bags

1 cup steamed almond milk

2 teaspoons sugar

Edible rose petals, to serve

## Directions

Dump all the ingredients (except the milk) into a large saucepan.

Cook the mixture for 5 minutes on a simmer.

Strain the hibiscus tea through a fine sieve and divide into serving mugs.

Add steamed almond milk to the tea.

Serve warm with rose petals on top.

Nutritional Values

Calories: 82

Total Fat: 14 g

Saturated Fat: 7 g

Cholesterol: 632 mg

Sodium: 497 mg

Total Carbs: 6 g

Fiber: 3 g

Sugar: 1 g

Protein: 5 g

## Turmeric Eggnog

Preparation Time: 10 minutes

Cooking Time: 0 minutes

Servings: 1

Ingredients

1 can light coconut milk

1 ½ cups water

3 pitted dates

1 teaspoon turmeric

1 teaspoon ground cinnamon

¼ teaspoon ground nutmeg

1/8 teaspoon ground allspice

1/8 teaspoon black pepper

1 tablespoon coconut oil

Directions

Dump all the eggnog ingredients into a blender jug.

Blend the eggnog mixture for 1 minute in the blender.

Garnish with nutmeg.

Serve.

Nutritional Values

Calories: 95

Total Fat: 1.1 g

Saturated Fat: 0.4 g

Cholesterol: 2 mg

Sodium: 84 mg

Total Carbs: 2.1 g

Sugar: 3.3 g

Fiber: 0.6 g

Protein: 2.4 g

## Conclusion

Those who follow a plant-based diet may need a little more carefully to prepare their meals. It can make all the difference to equip yourself with some dietary knowledge. Read our guides on vegetarian protein sources, where you can get vitamin B12 as well as the best plant sources of omega-3, may be useful.

When you change your diet drastically, starting gradually may be beneficial—maybe adding two or three meals based on plants, or days, a week. It helps the body to adapt to new foods and shifts in the percentage of certain nutrients, such as fiber. It also allows you to experiment with new foods over a period of time and create some store cupboard staples.

Weight loss is an almost certain result you will enjoy once you start the plant-based diet, but this is not the only benefit that you will enjoy. Think of all those activities you have always wanted to pursue but shelved because you simply had no energy left after your usual day's work.

Well, time to dust off those hobbies and the things you enjoy doing, because on the plant-based, you will have more energy for your daily work and play!

Something that many learn is that a diet is almost only as good as the number of recipes it has in its repertoire. The benefits of a particular diet may be numerous, but if you are forced to have the same stuff every breakfast, lunch and dinner, even the most avid supporter of the lot would probably have problems sustaining the diet. This is where I am most happy to say that the plant-based diet has quite some leeway for the concoction of various different recipes, and it is the purpose of this book to bring you some of the more delicious and easy-to-prepare meals for your gastronomic pleasure!

For the beginners as well as the adepts, the recipes contained within are created specifically to be appealing to your palate while not requiring you to literally spend the whole day in the kitchen! Concise and to the point, the recipes break down meal preparation requirements in a simple step by step format, easy for anyone to understand.

Don't forget to exercise. It has always been said that dieting is an effective way to lose weight. However, to keep the weight off, exercise is required. Many studies have shown that exercising while dieting is actually the best way to lose weight. Firstly, the diet becomes more effective and you lose weight faster if you exercise. But it also gets you in the habit of continuing your exercise when your diet is complete.